# General Book on Infectious Diseases

## By

## Venkataramana Rolla

**Table of Contents**

This book is a complete overview about infectious diseases. First volume will give you an idea about almost all types of infectious diseases, their root cause, symptoms and treatment options. This book is not a medical book and a regular ebook to offer general overview about all types of infectious diseases to a good extent. People often strained through many types of infectious diseases and some people dying through some of the dangerous diseases. This book is a tiny volume of effort to create awareness about various diseases.

Second volume of this book is aimed towards dangerous sexually transmitted diseases. These diseases are also explained to a good extent along with root cause and treatment option. Regular medical books will be little tough to understand for a common man and this book is written totally through a common man perspective to result into a great help and awareness.

## Infectious diseases start with "A"

**Abscess:** This abscess root cause is bacterial infection and it is a pus-containing inflammatory nodule. This pus is made develops through dead and live microorganisms. There is a chance for this abscess to grow into larger when bacteria win fight against the white cells. Generally, these Abscesses can be found within the soft tissue that is next to the skin of the groin area or armpit area. These will generally occupy a place, where lymph glands are commonly located in human body. The bacteria named, staphylococci are the major common cause for this abscess. Fungal infections very often transform into abscess too.

Abscess is generally diagnosed through sight and though MRI or CAT scans too. Antibiotics are usually ideal for treating Abscess. Bacterial infection and fungal agents control will always be quite effective through antibiotics. The linings of abscess always have scope to pass through blood and drainage tube arrangement can control this factor to a great extent. Genially, abscess will tend to heal well through simple drainage and drug treatment along with drainage can result into effective treatment.

**Acinetobacter:** This one belongs to the aerobic bacteria Neisseriaceae family. It is a genus and will not produce any spores and will not move too. These are very commonly seen in nature, but few members of this family will result into illness for humans.

**AIDS:** AIDS is scientifically termed as Acquired Immune Deficiency Syndrome. It is a most dangerous viral disease with no immunization. Cure is still on invention for this disease. Human immunity will face crippling situation trough this disease. The victim of this disease will fail to fight against all types of infections and eventually leads to few types of cancer conditions. The first case of AIDS was identified in the year 1980 and later recognized it as epidemic all over the world. The HUMAN IMMUNODEFICIENCY VIRUS is the main cause for the AIDS and this HIV virus is now widely popular as AIDS virus too. Infected individual body fluids will be seen completely occupied by this virus. This virus is rampant to spread through breast milk, semen, blood and vaginal discharge. White blood cells are always trying their level best to fight against this virus. AIDS will start to show impact over T Cells and these cells will start to die slowly due to the AIDS virus. HIV will completely invades these t Cells down the line after the infection.

HIV or AIDS diagnosis is generally determined through the blood test. There are confirmed chances of AIDS for an individual, when the T cells count found to be less than 200. This count is always above 440 in a healthy individual. It is pretty hard to identify any symptoms through AIDS during initial period and this initial period often takes years too. There is a chance for the infected individual to be symptoms free and healthy up to 8 years and in some cases up to 11 years too. There is no certain cure or treatment for AIDS and medications can help to extend the life of the individual to a certain period. Currently, drugs for AIDS treatment are antiviral and prophylactic for fighting against infection besides few additional drugs consumption to safeguard against cancer.

**Actinomycosis:** This is another bacterial infection through the Arachnia propionica or Actinomyces bacteria. This type of bacteria is commonly present in mouth and tonsils. This infection will result for an individual through the introduction to a broken tissue. There is a chance for these bacteria to transfer through the bite of human too. This infection generally affects jaw and mouth to result into swelling along with pain. Eventually, skin will witness tiny openings for the pus discharge. This pus will be in the form of yellow color granules.

Diagnosis of Actinomycosis generally confirmed through microorganisms presence. Pencillin is the effective treatment for all types of Actinomycosis. Severe infection conditions will require few months of treatment. There are few more antibiotics available to treat this disease besides the successful Pencillin. It is highly essential to have proper diet along with suitable surgical drainage procedure for the effective treatment of this disease.

**Adenovirus:** Some types of adenoviruses will attack animals only, but 2% of these viruses have tendency to show affect over humans' to result into illness for respiratory system through mild flu or pneumonia. Important part is that the virus will not fadeout after treating effectively illness and this virus will stay within tonsils lymph glands and adenoids. These viruses are definitely not latent as herpes, but reproduction activity will be there with slow and constant pacing. This virus was first found to be rampant during World War II in 1950 and there are few researches still indicating their presence in many of the adults all over the world.

**Aedes:** This is a mosquito seen very widely all over the tropical areas and subtropical areas. Some of the species of these mosquitoes are capable enough to transmit diseases and disease causing organisms into the humans. Very commonly seen diseases through this kind of transmission are Eastern Equine Encephalitis, Dengue fever, Yellow fever and St. Louis encephalitis.

**Aedes albopictus mosquito:** This mosquito is perfect carrier of dengue virus and widely called with other name as Asian Tiger too. This mosquito is found to be arrived to USA in the year 1995 and came to USA from Japan shipment that reached to Houston and Texas.

**Amebiasis:** This infection is also known as amoebic dysentery too. This infection is caused through a parasite within intestine or liver. His parasite is called as Entamoeba histolytica, which commonly resides within the human feces and intestine tract. This will be a serious infection for infants and for the adults that are with bad immune system. This is commonly seen with all humans, but more rampant with homosexual males. These parasites can stay within a human for years without showing any symptoms too.

The root cause for this infection could be due to the tainted food that is with protozoa. People that do not wash their hands after using the bathroom can infect the food to result into amebiasis. Human contact is also another reason for this disease through an infected individual. Anal intercourse also can result into this disease. The commonly associated symptoms with this disease are diarrhea, abdominal pain, tender liver, tender abdomen, and weight loss, and jaundice, loose stools in the morning, fatigue and anorexia. The mentioned symptoms will appear from few days to months after the infection. Some people will not be exposed too much with disease, but few will tend to experience liver abscess, when this parasite invades intestines.

Examination of tools is the perfect diagnosis for is disease. This examination will require fresh feces and multiple samples for the exact and correct diagnosis. This disease treatment is proven to be effective with Metronidazole. Hand washing with proper precautions is the perfect choice to prevent this disease.

**Amebic Abscess:** This Amebic Abscess will be resulted through a protozoan parasite known as Entamoeba hystolytica and this will collect pus within the liver. The symptoms associated with this infection are abdominal pain, diarrhea, vomiting sensation and nausea. The effective treatment for this infection is chloroquine and metronidazole.

**Amebic Carrier State:** This is a condition within human to carry amebic organisms with no sign of any symptom about the infection. A healthy carrier will have chance to turn into amebic infection down the line. This carrier is highly contagious and requires careful disposal of its feces.

**Aminoglycosides:** This one belongs to the family of antibiotics, which includes amikacin, streptomycin, gentamicin, kanamycin, neomycin and tobramycin. These are toxic drugs for nerve to result into kidney infection or damage.

**Amoeba (ameba):** This is a single cell parasite only can be seen through a microscope. It is a protozoan can turn into different shapes while moving through water world. Ameba is famous for cell reproduction at an amazing fast rate. It can produce thousands of its generations in a single day. Most of the cells are prone to die pretty soon and few species survived can be dangerous to the humans in many ways.

**Anaerobic Bactria Infections:** Anaerobic bacteria are that, which can survive without oxygen and Clostridium Botulinum is the perfect example in this context. These types of bacteria are present all over the nature and in the human body. These anaerobic organisms are capable enough to create Gangrene, Tetanus and Botulism.

**Anisakiasis:** It is a parasitic worm and food poison that is commonly seen in Japanese dish made out of raw fish and sushi. There are around ten cases every year within the USA and there is a chance for few cases undiagnosed too. Japanese consume raw fish very often and Anisakiasis is very rampant in japan due to this reason. There is a chance to diagnosis this disease as appendicitis or Cohn's disease or intestine cancer or peptic ulcer too. The parasitic worm

Anisakis is the major food source for some types of fishes such as whales and dolphins. So, raw fish eaten by people will have more chances to get attacked by tis disease. The Anisakiasis larvae are seen in sushi, ceviche, sashimi, raw herring, pacific salmon, cod, flounder, haddock, and monkfish and in fluke too.

The symptoms associated with this infection are nausea, severe pain and vomiting. Surgery is the perfect choice for this situation. The worm or worms' removal is the only left out choice and surgery is the best option.

There is a chance for the patient to cough up worm and diagnosis should be carried out through examining the worm. It is highly imperative for the physician to examine stomach inside and intestine inside, when there is no cough up of the worm. The worm has to be killed by the cook through cooking or through freezing the fish. This is the possible prevention for this infection.

**Anopheles mosquito:** This Anopheles mosquito is capable enough to transmit dangerous Malaria to the humans.

**Anthrax:** This is another dangerous bacterial infection, which affects the livestock, but chances are there to spread over humans too. This will result into some types of skin cancers, lung infections. The root cause of the Anthrax is Bacillus Anthracis bacteria. This Anthracis is capable enough to stay within pastures for a long duration successfully. Damp and warm weather will help these bacteria to grow into multiples rapidly. This disease is too dangerous for cattle, goats, sheep and their wool too. Also, these bacteria can contaminate their bones too. This Bacillus is not highly infectious with humans. There is a chance for pulmonary anthrax, when this bacteria breathed by human. Also, there is a chance for dangerous intestinal anthrax, when ate flesh of animals that were died through anthrax.

The symptoms through anthrax are itchy feeling, which can turn into blister down the line. This blister will turn into black scab that is surrounded by swelling tissue. Shivering along with chills will attack the infected individual subsequently. Also, there is a chance for the bacteria to move towards the lymph node too. There is a chance for blood poisoning, when bacteria enter into the human blood stream, which will result into anthrax meningitis or internal bleeding. This Anthrax is curable, when treated during early stages. High dosage of Pencillin is wise option for this treatment. Advanced stage of Anthrax cannot stand Pencillin and it will require a special vaccine to cure the infection.

**Antibacterial Drugs:** Antibacterial drugs are designated to treat some types of infections that are caused through bacteria. Actions of these drugs are almost similar to other antibiotics, but these are produced synthetically unlike antibiotics. Most of the antibacterial agents used in these drugs are sulfonamides. Most of the physicians will not prefer to differentiate antibacterial drugs with antibiotics.

**Antibiotic Drugs:** Antibiotic drugs are designated to treat infections that are resulted through bacteria, but made of fungi and molds. Antibiotics that of broad-spectrum meant for special treatment against wider range of bacteria and rest are designated for treating specific bacteria.

**Antidiarrheal Drugs:** This antidiarrheal drug is derived to treat or control the symptoms of the diarrhea. This drug will act in many different ways like absorbing water of the digestive tract, changes actions of the intestine, changes electrolyte transport, absorbs toxins, and many more.

**Antifungal or Antiyeast Drugs:** These drugs are available in the form of injections, oral pill or through used directly over the skin for treating yeasts or fungi. These drugs are capable enough to treat most types of Tinea, which includes jock itch, scalp ringworm and Athlete's foot. These are effective to treat Thrush and some more fungal infections like Cryptococcus.

**Antihelmintic Drugs:** These are group of drugs that are capable enough to treat worm infestations more effectively. Human intestine is always a harbor for many types of worms. This will be termed as worm burden basing on the worms parasite qualities. Here, these antihelmintic drugs will be a great help to get rid of these worms and to prevent the possibilities for the complications. These drugs will kill or paralyze the worms within the intestine in order to keep them away from gripping the walls of the intestine. Eventually, these worms will be eliminated through feces.

**Antimalarial Drugs:** This is a medicine to prevent and destroy plasmodia that can cause into Malaria. Nowadays, this Malaria causing bacteria is being quite resistant against the usual types of therapies and this is resulting into a severe pressure for the worldwide health.

**Antimicrobial Drugs:** Microorganisms growth will be destroyed with the help of these drugs.

**Antipyretic Drugs:** This is a drug derived to reduce the fever through controlling the temperature of the body. Aspirin is the best example of this drug beisdes other popular drugs such as acetaminophen and some more as ibuprofen.

**Antiseptic:** It is a germicide that is capable enough to control germs reproduction over the human skin or over the tissue. Microbes will be weakened through the application of antiseptic and will not kill them. Most of the healthcare antiseptics that are widely seen in soaps can help well to control the spreading f infection to a good extent. Generally, antiseptics will contain alcohol, iodine, chlorhexidine, hydrogen peroxide, hexachlorophene or some more.

**Antitoxin:** The toxin formed through the bacteria within the body can be successfully eradicated with the help of antitoxin. These antitoxins will generally contain an antibody to fight against the toxin resulted through the bacteria. Practically speaking, this antitoxin will neutralize the toxin that is released by the bacteria. These antitoxins are available in the form of injections and these will be injected into the muscle of the individual. Antivenin is a perfect example in this context, which is a perfect antitoxin derived to be a snakebite combat.

**Antitussive Drugs:** This antitussive drug is one to reduce the cough through controlling the activity of the cough at the brain and through suppressing the breathing. These drugs are combination of the nonnarcotic and narcotics to act suitably over the peripheral and central nervous system of the body. This will suppress the reflex of the cough to a great extent successfully. In fact, cough reflex is the major aspect to clear upper respiratory system of the body. Here, these antitussive drugs are not suggested using for the cough that is combined with mucus, which is known as productive cough condition. These antitussive drugs are majorly available in the form of syrup along with alcohol and an expectorant. These are also seen available in the form of capsules too along with mild pain killer and antihistamine.

**Antiserum:** This is a combination of antibodies of a specific germ and few of the specific antigens in the form of foreign invaders. Generally, antiserum comes with living things like viruses or few bacteria and this will be a perfect emergency treatment for an unvaccinated individual that has been a prey for a dangerous disease or infection. This antiserum will be developed from the animal blood or human blood that is immunized already for the protection against the organism. This antiserum is a perfect instant help to protect the individual from the microorganisms. This antiserum will not be a preventive measure against the disease or infection, but result into a great help for the immunization treatment for the infected victim.

**Antiviral Agents:** Antiviral agents are the drugs to treat or control viral infection. Complete eradication of virus is till unavailable for the people and cause of the illness can be controlled through the drugs. Here, it is quite imperative to mention that viruses live within cells and killing tis virus can result into damage for the host cell too. The fight to kill the viruses from the scientists is still under progress keeping in mind the host cell situation intact. Here, antiviral agents will be successful to control the viral replication and succeeds well to control their chemical process too, which is known as viral metabolism. Some of the latest antiviral agents are capable enough to control the virus from entering into the healthy cells too. However, it is highly important to mention that these antiviral agents will show some of the significant side effects and patients using these drugs should be monitored adequately.

**Arboviral Infections:** These arboviral infections are resulted through few number of viruses transmitting through arthropods like ticks and mosquitos. Common types of infections come under this category are Encephalitis, Encephalomyelitis, St. Louis Encephalitis, Eastern Equine Encephalitis, hemorrhagic fever, California Encephalitis and Rift Valley fever. The mentioned infections are generally rampant during warm weather conditions, when most of the dangerous insects are active. There are around 520 varieties of well-known arboviruses and 100 among them are dangerous for humans. Arboviral infections are possible with everyone and most susceptible are elderly and younger individuals. Infected mosquitoes will be the major root cause for these infections.

The common symptoms associated with this infection are varying quite significantly basing on the severity of the infection. Most of the infections will be seen with no symptoms. Some infections will have symptoms like light fever or headache. Here, severe infections can result into intense headache along with fever and disorientation. Some of the severe conditions can lead to coma, paralysis, convulsions, tremor or death too. Generally, symptoms will start to appear from 5 to 15 days after the infection. There is no specific treatment for this infection, but relief from the symptoms can be sought through drugs. Prevention of the aboviral infections or diseases can be initiated through insect repellents.

**Arenavirus:** The granular outer shape of the virus inherited them the name arenavirus, which means sand in Latin. This virus was first time identified in the year 1993 during the outbreak of Encephalitis in St. Louis. This virus is quite unusual and deadly for humans. Luckily, these virus types are restricted their parameter to certain geographic locations, but these contagious. So, requires utmost attention and prevention measures against this virus worldwide.

**Arthritis and Septic:** This is also known as infective arthritis and some people call it as pyogenic arthritis too. This is joint diseases resulted through bacterial invasion from the nearby wound. Blood infection can also turn into arthritis in some cases. Here, arthritis caused through the nearby infection can turn into septic arthritis to result into more complications. Symptoms associated with disease are pain; swelling and joints will turn into hot. Generally, tis disease diagnosis is made through the joint appearance and basing on the joint fluid, which will be drawn through a needle. Performing culture test is essential part of the diagnosis. Antibiotic drugs are the choicest treatment for this arthritis infection and septic arthritis. Some cases will require surgical cleansing of the infected joint too.

**Aspergillosis:** This is a very rare type of infection, which affects badly the ear or some other organ with fungus. Some cases, this will affect mucous membranes of nose or the urethra or some of the internal organs like kidneys, lungs, and liver. This infection got more chances to spread all over the body and this will be rampant with the people that are with impaired immune condition. Amphotericin B will be suggested using for treating systemic aspergillosis. Acute conditions will be ideal to treat through steroids.

**Aspergillus:** This is fungi to cause some respiratory infections for humans. This fungus is very commonly seen in soil. Most of the allergic reactions will be the damage through these fungi.

**Athlete's Foot:** This is a fungal condition for the skin between toes. Very commonly affects at fourth and fifth toes. It will result into itch, crack, and peel besides diffuse scaling along with redness over sides and soles. This will generally happen through shoe wearing and its sweating process. This is known as Athlete's foot and this infection will last until the lesions will heal properly well. Dermatophytes are the root cause for the Athlete's Foot infection. The two main Dermatophytes that are reason for Athlete's Foot are T. mentagrophytes and Trichophton rubrum. There is a chance for this infection to transmit through locker rooms, towels sharing, shoes sharing and through showers.

Symptoms associated with this infection are cracking, and scaling of the skin at the toes area, sides of feet and itchy and peeling skin all over the feet. Also, there is a chance for little water blisters within toes and these can result into spreading the infection too. Bad odor is another symptom commonly associated with this infection. Diagnosis of this infection can be completed through microscope the affected scraping for ascertain the fungal characteristics. There is a chance for this infection to clear up on own, but treatment will always be ideal. There are many over the counter fungicide sprays available to treat this Athlete's Foot effectively. Good hygiene is the better choice to prevent this Athlete's foot. It is a good option to disinfect your shower floors and locker room to prevent this infection successfully.

**Avian Flu:** Avian flu is widely known as "bird-flu" too. Avian-flu virus is the root cause for this disease. This virus travels successfully from chickens to humans. This flu virus is totally away from other flu viruses that are commonly result into chill and fever. It will attack directly over the respiratory system and this will result into severe hemorrhage for every tissue of the body including brain. This virus is scientifically termed as "H5 flu" as it carries H5 variation of H gene. This H gene is a variation, which is lethal in chickens. Initially, this disease started in Hong Kong for the people that were in direct contact with poultries and later spread all over Hong Kong through contact. The total epidemic was stopped by the Hong Kong government through killing all chickens in Hong Kong, but scientists still fear that this virus could successfully exchange genetics with other common flu virus.

## Infectious Diseases Start with "B"

**Babesiosis:** This babesiosis is a fatal disease caused through microorganisms that are purely tick-borne. These microorganisms are almost similar to Lyme disease and HGE. This disease is very much prone with immune impaired elder individuals and this is also known as Nantucket fever too. This disease is caused through the protozoa that are almost similar Malaria causing species. Tick bites will be the major reason for this disease. Contaminated blood transfusion is another reason for this disease. Symptoms associated with this disease are mild illness and some more. These symptoms will start to appear over the infected individual within one to twelve months duration. It can be identified through fever, hemolytic anemia, fatigue, and all these symptoms will last for few days to few months. There is a chance for no symptoms with few infected individuals too. Molecular test is the wise option to diagnosis this disease. There is no standardized treatment for this disease, but combination of antimalarial drug and an antibiotic can offer reasonable relief for the infected individual. This can be prevented through tick repellents and controlling the rodents all around your home.

**Bacillary Angiomatosis:** This is another dangerous infectious disease and this will result into formation of tumor kind masses through growing blood vessels within bones, skin and liver. The resulted tumor like masses will almost look like Kaposi's sarcoma.

**Bacillus:** This is a large genus bacterium, which is gram-positive and spore-bearing too. This is comprised of 33 species and three among them are diseases causing species. These are commonly seen in air and soil and root cause for many different varieties of diseases. Some of the best examples will be Anthrax and food poisoning. These are commonly feed over dead matter to result into food spoilage.

**Bacillus Anthracis:** This is Anthrax causing gram-positive bacterium. This bacterium is dangerous for sheep and cattle. This bacterial will result into pulmonary anthrax though inhaling the spores and these spores are capable enough to survive for years together in wool and in hides.

**Bacillus Polymyxa:** This one belongs to the Bacillus species and lives in soil. It is the major source for the polymyxin group of antibiotics too.

**Bacillus Subtilis:** This one also belongs to the Bacillus species and it will cause conjunctivitis for humans. This is also used widely for the production of antibiotic bacitracin.

**Bacteremia:** This bacteremia is an invasion into the blood stream. This will cause skin infection, strep throat and tonsillitis. This infection got more chances to spread through the infected blood stream towards other areas of the human body. This spreading will result into abscesses, heart inflammation, peritonitis, and meningitis. This bacteremia can also cause circulatory collapse or general illness along with severe fever, or some organ failure.

**Bacteria:** These are microbes, which are not organized well into a cell nucleus similar to animals and plants. Here, some bacteria are capable enough to make own food and few are purely dependent over other organisms for their food needs. Some type of bacteria can make own food and live as parasites too on other organisms. Some type of bacteria require air to survive as rest will survive without air successfully too. Some bacteria can move on own and few cannot move at all. These bacteria can be seen in different shapes, colors and sizes. It is highly imperative to mention that all bacteria not harmful as there are few helpful bacteria among them. There are more than 400 varieties of bacteria that help well for the digestion system of the human. There are many disease causing bacteria too existent and these disease causing bacteria is nowadays resulting into more resistant towards the doctor prescribed antibiotics too. Nowadays, 60% of the infections that are hospitalizing humans are due to the drug-resistant bacteria.

**Bacterial Infections:** Bacterial infections are the most threatening infectious diseases in this world. Some of those are bacterial meningitis, gonorrhea, tuberculosis, bacterial pneumonia, whooping cough, typhoid and many more.

**Bactericide:** this bactericide is a substance that is capable enough to kill bacteria.

**Bang's disease:** This Bang's disease is other name for the Brucellosis.

**Bartonella:** This is another gram-negative small genus belongs to coccobacilli, which is capable enough to infect red blood cells. This can also infect liver, spleen and lymph nodes too.

**Bartonellosis:** This is an acute bacterial infection caused through the bite of a sand-fly. This sand-fly bite risk is possible in Southwest Colombia mountain valleys and in Peru. This sand-fly carries successfully bacterium that is capable enough to result into disease. This sand-fly often feeds between dusk and dawn and during this period transmission will have more possibilities for the bartonellosis. The some of the symptoms associated with bartonellosis are veruga peruana and oroya fever. The oroya fever symptoms will start to appear within three weeks after the sand-fly bite. This fever will be accompanied along with headache, joints and bones aching. This will be followed by the severe anemia along with swollen lymph nodes. This disease will last up to six weeks period, but result into fatal in some cases. Veruga peruana can be identified through nodules appearance over face and limbs, which will bleed regularly. This condition will last up to a year. The complete healing will end up with scarring.

Generally, ampicillin or chloramphenicol are the wise treatment options for the bartonellosis and Pencillin, streptomycin and tetracycline can also prove to be fine for the this disease. Prevention of this disease is only through avoiding the sand-fly bite.

**Blastomycosis:** This blastomycosis is a mild and self-limiting type yeast infection. This infection will start initially in lungs and eventually spreads other areas of the body. It will be more dangerous, when infection spreads to bones and skin. Children and adult aged between forty and sixty are more prone for this infection. This disease is also known as Gilchrist's disease or Chicago disease or as North American blastomycosis too. The root cause of this disease is blastomyces dermatiidis yeast, which is almost similar to Cryptococcus neoformans or Coccidioides immitis.

Symptoms associated with this disease are inflammation, which normally varies basing on its location on the body. There is a possibility for the widespread inflammation in lungs along with small signs of abscesses. The popular drug Amphotericin B is the wise choice for this disease. Also, you can consider hydroxystilbamidine, when disease is affecting skin. There is a good chance for successful results with itraconazole and ketaconazole too.

**Blepharitis:** This is an infection identified through the chronic inflammation for long duration for eyelids and eyelashes. This is a common infection for age group humans. You can identify this infection through the red colored scaly irritated skin over the edges of eye lids. Sometimes, eyelids' glands will produce excess oil and this will result into blepharitis and poor hygiene lids are also another reason. Scalp dandruff is another reason for this infection and this will result into seborrheic blepharitis.

The symptoms associated with the blepharitis are greasy flakes or scaling all over eyelashes base along with mild redness of eyelid. There is a chance for tissue roughness, which can create lines within the eyelids through the seborrheic blepharitis. Styes may also appear through the acute eyelids infection too. This is generally not a serious infection and scaling can be controlled successfully with the help of moistened cotton through warm water. Definitely, recurring inflammation deserves medical treatment through a physician. There is a chance for severe cases to affect cornea too.

**Boil:** This infection normally appears at moist areas like backside of neck, groin and armpits. These boils are generally inflammatory and pus-filled portion of skin and very commonly seen as a hair follicle infection. These boils will develop through bacterium infection known as Staphyloccus aureus. This will generally invades entire body through a break over the skin, when this infection blocked oil gland or a hair follicle. This boil will generally starts with red lump that swells along with pain and pus. Eventually, this boil will turn into a round bump with yellow color tip. It will erupt down the line at one point of time to fade away. This boils will reappear with the individuals that are with low body resistance or diabetes.

Treatment for boils is through hot compress for a period of twenty minutes in every 2 hours. Generally, a boil will take one week time to break and proper cleaning is essential to control the infection spreading to other areas of the body. It is a good idea to consult physician for antibiotics, when the boils are large and more painful.

**Bordetella:** This is a gram-negative genus and some species in it can cause respiratory disease for humans.

**Bordetella Pertussis:** This is small gram-negative anaerobic bacteria to cause whooping cough in humans. This is very common infection to be seen all over the world. All of other species in Bordetella genus will also cause disease that is almost similar to whooping cough.

This infection is contagious through contact. This infection generally strikes during childhood and this infection is resulting into many infant deaths all over the world. In the year 1940, a vaccine was developed for this infection against the bacteria.

**Borna Disease Virus (BDV):** This is a virus to cause neurological disease and behavior disruptions in animals and humans. Depression can trigger in humans through this infection. This is a single-stranded RNA virus, which is capable enough to spread persistent infection keeping the host cell intact. This BDV creates neurological symptoms in animals and these symptoms will be seen as manic-depression with humans, when affected. This BDV infects cells within the limbic system in order to result into many psychiatric disorders in humans.

**Botulism:** The food-borne illness is known as botulism infectious disease. This infection involves production of toxin by bacteria that is deadly and rare. This botulism appeared in infants of one year old is known as "infant botulism" infectious disease. Scientifically, it is a poisoning and cannot be termed as an infectious disease. This is not an infection that can be transmitted to others. This botulism is a toxin that is a type of neurotoxin that normally attaches to nerves and succeeds in blocking the messages that were sent muscles. Symptoms will appear within twelve to twenty-six hours and first sign would be muscle weakness. This leads to double vision eventually. Victim will start witness trouble with speaking and swallowing due to the muscle paralysis. There are some more symptoms added to this condition with nausea, diarrhea, vomiting, , stomach cramps and some more.

This can be diagnosed through the presence of toxin within the food, stool and blood. The treatment will require instant administration of antitoxin, which can stop the damages to health including death. Canned food is often reason for the botulism and this can be prevented through boiling the canned food at 100 degrees C for every minute.

**Botulism, Infant:** This infant botulism is generally seen with babies below 6 months age and this is less serious infection unlike with adults' botulism. Botulism in adults and infants caused due to the toxins released by bacteria. Clostridium botulinum is the toxin that results into botulism. A baby with infant botulism will not ingest toxin and the spores of botulism will reproduce toxin within digestive system of the infected infant, which will travel successfully to the baby's nerve cells. Hospital treatment can help these babies to recover well and fast.

This infant botulism is a rare disease tough to trace as spores got more chances to survive for a longer duration. Commercial honey in the market can contain these botulism spores to result into infant botulism for infants. There is a chance for the dark and light corn syrup too contain these bacteria. The infant infected will excrete this toxin through feces, but this infection will not pass to others. The symptoms associated are flaccidity for facial muscle, constipation, irritability, floppy arms, sucking issues and lethargy. Sudden Infant Death Syndrome is the serious complication associated with this infection. Treatment through antitoxin is not ideal for infants and antibiotics will be the left out possible option to treat infant botulism. Severe cases may deserve breathing assistance and recovery will be completely slow process in this treatment.

**Bovine Spongiform Encephalopathy:** The medical name of this disease is Mad Cow Disease. This is an infectious disease normally seen in cows and now emerged in the humans too. BSE first identified in the year 1986 in Britain. This disease was transmitted to humans through the contaminated meat and bone.

**Brain Abscess:** This infection is commonly seen in temporal and frontal lobes and this will be transmitted from other body parts like sinuses. Infection in the bones, infection in the heart or brain outside nervous system infection also can result into brain abscess too. 10% brain abscess cases can be fatal and rest will experience little brain function issues. The common complication associated with this infection is seizure disorder. Vomiting, headache and sleepiness are the common symptoms associated with this infection. Severe state can lead to vision problem along with seizures and fever. There is a chance for speech problems and partial paralysis too. Scanning only can diagnosis this problem and CT or MRI is suggested by the doctors to prove the infection. High dose of antibiotics are required to treat this problem. Surgery will be the ultimate option, which will access abscess through a hole created in the skull.

**Brazilian Purpuric Fever:** This is a dangerous systematic illness resulted through bacterial infection. This disease was first identified in Brazil in the year 1984. So far, there were no cases identified with this disease other than southern Brazil. This BPF is very much related to the Haemophilus aegyptius and untreated infection will be fatal through spreading to the skin through the released toxins. Eye infection is the first symptom arrives with this disease. Eventually, bacteria will spread all over the body to result into bleeding skin and fever.

Antibiotics are the available option to treat this disease and antibiotics usage before to skin bleeding can prevent the progressing infection to a great extent.

**Breast Cancer and Virus:** Some of the latest researches are informing that the breast cancer is caused through a virus. Here, it is quite imperative to mention that the cancerous breast cell very often seen with genetic sequence that is almost similar to some of the infectious virus that causes mammary tumors. The research findings are still under scanner for the valid conclusive proof.

**Bronchiolitis:** This is a viral infection generated in the lungs' airways and this is capable enough affect infants and children. Here, smaller airways that are branching off bronchial tubes will turn into inflamed and this is mainly due to the Respiratory Syncytial Virus. Shortness of breath cough and purple-blue skin are the common symptoms seen with this infection. Very often, a physician can hear some bubbling noise within the lungs of the infected individual too. It is highly imperative to consult a physician, when an infant or young child is suffering from worse cough and cold. Hospitalization is essential treatment for a young child that is suffering from severe bronchiolitis. Some of the Corticosteroid drugs and antibiotics will result into in vain for this infection treatment. Here, prescribed antibiotics will be a help to control secondary bacterium infection. Sometimes suffering child may require artificial ventilation too.

**Bronchitis:** This is another viral infection to result into inflammation for airways that are connected to the windpipe of lungs, which will result into continuous cough along with sputum or phlegm. This will be rampant during winter with smokers, people with lung issues, children and elderly. This bronchitis can be seen in the form of acute and chronic conditions. Here, acute condition is viral infection caused due to air pollution. Bacterial infection also can result into acute bronchitis and this will be seen attacking during winter. Chronic bronchitis is a result through smoking. This smoking causes reasonable stimulation for the mucus production.

The symptoms associated with the bronchitis are similar with acute and chronic conditions. The symptoms will start to appear, when bronchial tubes swelled and congested. Here, infected individual will experience breathlessness, wheezing, phlegm in green or yellow shade and continuous cough. Lungs humidification is the necessary treatment for this issue and humidifies the lungs with steam inhaling or with a humidifier. Generally, acute bronchitis will clean up on own. Chronic bronchitis will require bronchodilator inhaler, which can help to offer relief from the breathlessness.

**Brucella:** This is gram-negative spherical genus and rod like parasite bacteria. This bacteria can cause Brucellosis in humans and causes contagious abortion for animals.

**Brucellosis:** This is another chronic bacterial infectious disease transmitted through farm animals. This virus is capable enough to attack human organs and other name for this infection is undulant fever. This disease is generally caused through several types of bacteria species that belongs to Brucella genus. This disease will cause intermittent fevers, but not a fatal one. Symptoms will take five to thirty days to appear over the infected individual. Blood test only can diagnosis this infection. It requires prolonged treatment with the help of antibiotics.

Sulfonamides will be effective for treating this problem. Immunizing the livestock will be the possible prevention measure against this infection.

**Bunyavirus:** This is mosquito borne virus that can infect humans to cause into California Encephalitis, Rift Valley Fever and some more. The common symptoms associated with this infection are facial pain, fever, rashes, headache and weakness.

## Infectious Diseases Starts with "C"

**Campylobacter:** This is a bacteria reason for the 14% of diarrhea cases. This bacterium was first time found in the year 1909 and named as Vibrio fetus. This bacterium is capable enough to survive successfully at the body temperature and poultry, pets, horses and cattle. There are four different types of organisms that can infect intestine and this is one among those four. Tainted food is the major source to ingest these organisms in the human body. Many unhygienic conditions and wrong cooking habits can also be a reason for this infection.

**Campylobacteriosis:** This is food-borne illness identified in the year 1970. This infection will leads to gastroenteritis. There are wide varieties of forms for this campylobacter and most common form is campylobacter jejuni. This is the main reason for the 995 of camylobacter infections. Contaminated water and food can turn into campylobacteriosis. This is capable enough to survive through cooked food like chicken, beef, lamb and pork. It can also survive well in mail and water too. Diarrhea affected pets like cats and dogs are the perfect carriers of this disease to young children. The symptoms will start to appear within ten days after the infection and it will last up to ten days too. Abdominal pain, vomiting and nausea are the common symptoms through this infection. Stool testing in lab is the perfect diagnosis procedure for this infection. Symptoms can be controlled quickly through consuming antibiotics in the initial stage. Antibiotics also will result into a great help to shorten the infection too. There is a chance for this infection to turn into complication as paralyzed neurologic illness. This complication is possible only with less percentage infected individuals.

**Campylobacter Jejuni:** This is a slender bacterium belongs to Campylobacter genus. This bacterium is the major reason for bacterial diarrhea and it will be almost like a combination of Shigella and Salmonella. There is no chance for healthy humans to carry this bacterium, but birds, cattle, chickens and flies are possible carriers.

**Candida Albicans:** This is yeast commonly found in human body and results into infection called as candidiasis. This is yeast more often seen in vagina or within the mucous membranes. Other name for this infection is moniliasis. This candidiasis or Thrush causes cottage cheese kind patches within the mouth and it is common AIDS sign for young adults.

**Candida Lusitaniae Infection:** This is a rare human pathogen that can form into fungal infection. Generally, this will result into infection in lung, meninges, kidney, and lower part of urinary tract, skin, gastrointestinal tract, soft tissue and bone. This C. Lusitaniae infection generally starts within throat or within gastrointestinal tract. Blood test only can reveal the presence of this infection for humans. This is a pathogen and it is quite resistant to amphotericin B. So, add flucytosine along with other popular antifungal drugs. So far, 30% infected individuals died due to this infection.

**Canker Sore:** his is a tiny painful ulcer, develops within mouth, or over lip or below to the tongue. Generally, this will heal on own without any treatment. This is a gray center tiny oval ulcer surrounds with red halo. This will last almost for two weeks. These are little larger than the fever sores in size. There are many over the counter drugs available to treat canker sore, but consider medication that is with carbamide peroxide for effective results.

**Carbuncle:** This carbuncle is a pus-filled boils cluster that is infected through bacteria. This kind of infection is very commonly seen neck back and over buttocks. These carbuncles are generally resulted through staphylococcus aureus bacterium. This infection starts with a single boil and spreads into cluster. Treatment for this carbuncle will be ideal through oral drugs and some of the tropical antibiotics. Hot compress also works fine against this infection.

**Carditis:** Heart muscles inflammation is caused in general through viral infection. This is known as carditis and one layer of the heart generally exposed to this infection. Heart beat will be irregular through this infection besides some more symptoms like circulatory failure, chest pain, and sometimes heart structure can damage to a certain extent too. This carditis can be seen in multiple forms as endocarditis, myocarditis, and pericarditis.

**Cats and Infectious Disease:** many varieties of multi-drug resistant bacterium can be widespread through cats. The salmonella bacteria in cats can result into 110 varieties of infections for humans.

**Cat-Scratch Disease (CSD):** A scratch or bite from your kitten or cat can result into mild illness and this is mainly due to the bacterium called as Bartonella henselae. This cat-scratch disease can result into few dangerous problems for healthy people. Importantly, immune system weakens through this disease and sometimes can turn into life threatening health issue too. The symptoms associated with CSD are almost like Tuberculosis and this will appear after two weeks to the scratch or bite. A round lump in red color can be witnessed at the infected area along with two or more lymph nodes with swelling. Fever will add up to these symptoms along with headache, malaise, rash and some more. Symptoms only can indicate the disease and there is no special diagnosis procedure for it. Currently, antibiotics are not available for CSD, but some pain killers will be prescribed for children that are with pain due to swelling lymph nodes.

**Cellulitis:** This is a bacterial infection for the skin along with underneath tissue. Failing to treat this infection can result into Septic Shock and bacteremia. The facial cellulitis will have chances to spread to brain and eyes. Generally, this cellulitis will be caused through B-hemolytic streptococci bacteria. The affected portion will normally experience red, hot and tender condition. There is a chance for fever, lymph glands swelling, and chills. Diagnosis through culture is tough for this infection, but infection can be easily located in blood. This infection commonly tends resolve on own spontaneously. Aspirin along with cold compress can bring reasonable relief for the infected victim.

**Cereus:** It is a variety of food poisoning happens through the bacillus cereus bacterium. This bacterium successfully multiplies within raw food at the room temperature. The toxins produced by the B. Cereus bacteria can be found very commonly in fried or steamed rice. This food poisoning can be seen in two different varieties. The first variety can be seen in food that is with less incubation period. The second variety is almost same like C. perfringens poisoning. There is no perfect cure for this infection, but available drugs can offer reasonable comfort for the victim.

**Chagas Disease:** This is another parasitic disease widely popular as American Trypanosomiasis. This infection generally comes through insect bites that suck blood. Also, there is a chance for this disease through blood transfusion too. This disease is generally happens through single-cell parasite called Trypanosoma cruzi. This disease can be seen in acute and chronic form with the infected individuals. This disease is more rampant in children than adults. Symptoms will be enlarged spleen, weakness, fever, lymph nodes, face and legs swelling and quite rapid heartbeat. Chronic illness doesn't have treatment, but acute infection can be treated successfully with Nifurtimox from CDC.

**Chagres Fever:** This Chagres fever is an abovirus infection. This is generally transmitted through sand-fly bite in humans. Muscle pain, fever and headache are common symptoms with this disease. Bed rest is the ideal treatment for this infection along with consuming more fluids and pain killers.

**Chancroid:** This is a rare STD, but seen its comeback since 1980. This Chancroid is caused through Hemophilus ducreyi bacterium. This bacterium generally transmitted draining sores of the infected individual. Symptoms will appear within a week after the infection. It is highly essential to consume antibiotics by both partners like erythromycin or azithromycin. The ceftriaxone shot can cure this infection successfully within a week. There is a chance for the chancroid to turn into ulcer, when untreated.

**Chicken pox (varicella):** this is a childhood infectious disease and seen very commonly during spring and winter. Chicken pox virus generally stays within the victim in latent phase within nerves and spinal cord lower portion. If this virus reactivated, then it will turn into shingles. This virus caused through airborne droplets will be more contagious. This virus will have up to 23 days of incubation period. Generally, red itchy rash spot will develop and it will turn into blister with fluids within a short duration of hours. New spots will start to appear within 7 days. Rest is the best treatment for the children with chicken pox. Victim will recover successfully within ten days.

**Chiggers:** Chiggers are the larva form of Trombicula mites and this will cause irritation and itching for skin. These are widely popular as harvest mites too. The swelling caused through chiggers can turn into blisters and these blisters can stay for weeks.

**Chikungunya Fever:** This is another dangerous infectious disease and his virus is very commonly found in central Africa, southeastern Asia and southwestern Africa. The chikungunya virus generally carried through A. aegypti mosquitos and this will transmit through this mosquito bite to humans. Fever along with chills; headache, vomiting and nausea are symptoms for this disease. In fact, specific treatment is not available for this disease, but pain killers can help to control the fever and other symptoms to a good extent.

**Chlamydia:** This is very common STD and chlamydia organisms will cause this infection to humans. This chlamydia is a bacterium, but looks almost like virus. This disease will transmit through sexual intercourse with infected individual. Also, this will transmit through birth too. Symptoms will include pain while urinating and discharge from private parts. Culture can reveal this disease quite easily and untreated infection can lead to infected tubes in female and chances for uterus lining infection too. Many types of antibiotics are available to treat this issue.

**Chlamydia Pneumonia Infection:** Chlamydia pneumonia infection is caused through the some types of chlamydia organism to result into respiratory illness, heart diseases, heart attack and some more. This organism will spread quite fast via person to person through cough or through the sneeze. Symptoms will appear after 21 days of infection and diagnosis has to be carried out through lab tests. Currently, azithromycin and clarithromycin are treating this problem perfectly well.

**Chlamydia Psittaci Infection:** This infection causes through an organism that will infect birds to result into rare variety of pneumonia. This rare type of pneumonia in humans is called as psittacosis. Generally, this infection is transmitted through breathing droplets of bacterium from the birds that were infected by the organism. Symptoms will appear between 6 and 19 days after infection exposure with birds. Flu kind of illness will surrounds the victim along with chills and fever, headache, rash, facial pain and some more. Blood test is the best diagnosis procedure to find out the presence of this infection. Tetracycline is the perfect treatment for this infection for total 3 weeks.

**Chlamydia Trachomatis:** This is a serious, but curable infection. This infection can result into some types of urinary tract infections in both genders. This also can result into ectopic pregnancy or pelvic inflammatory disease too. There are few antibiotics available to treat this problem to a good extent. This is a STD and prevention of this disease is very much possible through using condom.

**Cholera:** Cholera is an infection that infects small intestine in humans. This will turn into rapid dehydration, when failed to treat in time. Fluids are the best option to improve the recovery of the victims. Cholera is caused through Vibrio cholerae bacterium. This is another dangerous and contagious infection with more chances to transmit to others. A positive stool culture can reveal cholera presence for a patient. This will turn into complicate watery diarrhea, when not treated properly. Replacing lost fluids is the best treatment for cholera. Here, some of the antibiotics can help to shorten the diarrhea period infection to a great extent.

**Chromomycosis:** This is one of the dangerous chronic and invasive fungal infections. Generally, it will attack the top two layers of skin over legs and feet. This infection caused through molds very commonly seen in soil. Manual labors are very much prone to this disease. The symptoms are warty nodule along with itchy and watery nature. Initially, it will appear as a red dull lesion. Bed rest along with elevation of infected portion is the best treatment option for this problem. Here, usage of antibiotics can control successfully the secondary infection stage. Chronic infection that is lasting for years can involve amputation.

**Chronic Fatigue Syndrome:** This is a disease associated with group of symptoms such as weakness, fatigue, poor memory, and some more. This disease is also known as "yippie flu" too. Still the exact root cause of this problem uncertain. Persistent fatigue that is tough to explain is the major symptom of this disease. There are some more symptoms associated with this disease as sore throat, lack of concentration and memory, muscle pain, headache, malaise, tender lymph nodes, joint pain and some more. There is no specific treatment for this problem, but anti-inflammatory drugs can help to gain relief against pains.

**Ciguatera:** This is very common type clinical syndrome caused through the consumption of tropical reef fish. This Ciguatera can happen through eating any of 300 species of fishes that are with ciguatoxin. There will be neurologic and stomach symptoms with this disease. Also, victims will experience sensory reversal issues too. Antidotes are the wise option to treat ciguatera effectively.

**Clonorchiasis:** This is an infection caused through parasite flatworms that are generally present within raw fresh water fish or improper cooked fish. This parasite will not be seen in saltwater fishes. Fatigue, abdominal pain and fever are common symptoms associated with this disease. Proper cooking of freshwater fish is essential to prevent this disease.

**Clostridium:** This is another spore generating bacteria commonly seen in earth all over the world. Some of these bacteria forms can be seen intestines. These are capable enough to poison the food and results into wound infection too.

**Clostridium Difficile:** this is another bacterium species that generates two different types of toxins to result into pseudomembranous colitis. Eradication of these bacteria is highly tough and threatens hospitals to a great extent. These spores are capable enough to survive over the hospital floors for many months. Antibiotics consumption should be stopped for the victims of this infection. It is ideal to consider metronidazole or vancomycin.

**Clostridium Perfringens Infection:** This is another food-borne mild illness through toxin multiplication from Clostridium perfringens type A Bacterium. This type of bacteria generally found in animal and human feces and also found in water and soil too. These bacteria are normally seen in uncooked meat too. Undercooked meat is the major source for producing toxin by this organism. These bacteria normally seen in spore form cannot be killed through cooking. The illness through this infection will happen within 9 to 24 hours after the consumption. These bacteria can grow over culture plate in lab and stool sample can detect this bacteria presence successfully. Technically, this cannot be termed as an infection and it is intoxication. Antibiotic will fail to cure this issue. Fluid losses replacement is the ideal treatment for this problem. Dehydration situation should be dealt through a doctor.

**Clostridium Tetani:** This tetanus creating bacteria belongs to the Clostridium genus. These bacteria found in soil and gains entry into the human body through wounds and deep puncture type cuts. These bacteria will be quite active over the decomposed tissue and lets the toxin travel directly into the nervous system and later into spine. This will trigger spasm to activate the syndrome known as "lockjaw".

**Coccidiides Immitis:** This is an infectious fungal seen in the form of spores and it can cause chronic or acute illness known as coccidioidomycosis.

**Coccidioidomycosis:** This is also known as valley fever, which is infectious fungal disease. This will cause through inhaling bacteria spores. The results can be acute or chronic illness for the victim. The bacteria spores are perfect windborne particles to result into instant disease. This will infect lungs. Initial stage of the illness will resemble like flu. Fever, chills, sweating, headache, fatigue and cough are common symptoms of this disease. The diagnosis can be carried out through identifying fungus in sputum or through body fluid or through tissue. Valley fever generally subside on own, but disease spread to other body parts will require medical attention. The common antibiotics suitable for this valley fever are itraconazole, fluconazole and ketoconazole.

**Cold, Common:** Cold is generally happened through one of the 200 varieties of viruses, which will affect the upper respiratory into infection. Cold season is commonly the time to suffer this common cold by all. The cold attack during spring can be caused through any one of the 100 different varieties of rhinovirus. Cold virus cannot travel far through air. Congested nose is the pretty common symptom for cold besides sneezing, sore throat, headache, cough low fever, runny eyes and some more. In fact, there is no cure for cold, but antibiotics are available to reduce the symptoms.

**Cold Sore:** This is also known as "fever blister" and it can be seen as a tiny skin blister. These are generally transmitted during childhood and these are pretty common too. These are completely harmless, but little painful. These are almost similar to the canker sores. These are caused through Herpes Simplex virus. This is more contagious virus. Kissing can transmit this disease quite faster. Touching blisters can also transmit this disease to others. Generally, cold sores will appear before the age of 10 with completes nil symptoms. Subsequent outbreak will signal lips tingling, which follows water-filled blisters. This blister will burst and disappear soon. Here, the virus will be dormant within the nerve cell and there is a more chance for reactivation anytime. There is no treatment for cold sores, but sore should always be kept dry and clean.

**Coliform Count:** This is a procedure to find out the fecal coliform level within water. This count will include all varieties of coliform bacterium strains.

**Communicable/Contagious Disease:** A disease that is communicable or contagious through various form including touching is termed as a disease. Here, controlling the communicable disease is mainly depends over the organism s observation. This will reveal the total procedure that organisms are practicing to transmit a disease.

**Condylomata Acuminata:** this is a wart very common to happen near genitals. This kind of infection will generally spread through sexual contact. This infection in human is caused by papillomavirus. The common symptom for this disease is moist genital folds along with creases. There is no specific treatment for these warts as Papillomavirus is hard to eradicate and it survived with laser treatment too. This most area can be treated effectively with the help of podophyllin chemical.

**Congenital Infectious Disease:** This is a disease present in infant before to birth or acquired while passing through birth canal. There is a huge chance for many varieties of bacteria, microorganisms and viruses to come in contact with placenta from mother blood into the infant body. Here, effect of the microorganism will be mainly dependent over the pregnancy stage, where infection initiated.

**Congo Fever (Congo-Crimean hemorrhagic fever):** It is an infectious disease caused through the tick bite. This will result into fever along with bleeding from the skin and mucous membranes. This viral infection generally transmitted to humans via tick. The genus Hyalomma is the reason for this infectious disease. Symptoms will be visible within 2 to 7 days after the infection. This will associate with fever, muscle pains, chills, vomiting and headache. Testing blood in the laboratory can reveal the presence of disease. There is no cure for this disease and treatment is available to control the symptoms.

**Conjunctivitis:** medical name for this disease is "pink eye" and it is a common childhood infection. This conjunctivitis caused through staphylococci bacteria and transmitted successfully through eye contact. Itchy red eye is the common symptom besides pain, discharge, scratchy and photophobia. There are antibiotic eye drops to treat this disease and ointment will be a wise choice, when suspected bacterial infection.

**Coronavirus:** Coronavirus is reason for simple respiratory issues and common cold. Fatal illness will never develop in humans through this virus. These viruses will capable enough to offer symptoms to their victims within three days. These symptoms will stay for a period of one week. Very common problem with this virus is nasal congestion and there is a chance to re-attack the victim again and again by the virus too.

**Corticosteroid Drugs:** These are highly extreme drug group and very often termed as steroids. These are almost similar to natural corticosteroid hormones that are produced successfully by the adrenal glands. These drugs are derived to fight against the different types of inflammatory conditions.

**Corynebacterium Diphtheriae:** This is Diphtheria causing bacteria generally stays within mouth, nose, and throat of the infected person. This bacterium successfully transmits to other through cough, contact, sneeze, nose discharge, skin, throat, lesions and eyes. This is a common throat disease similar to Strep Throat.

**Cowpox:** This is an infection generally affects cows through Vaccinia virus. This Vaccinia virus is used generally as a vaccine for small pox for humans.

**Coxiella Burnetti:** Rickettsia is another name for the Coxiella burnetti and this organism will cause fever in humans.

**Coxsackievirus:** This is an enterovirus with more than 30 varieties in it. This will affect children with different symptoms during warm weather conditions. This germ is almost looks like Polio virus. This virus can cause herpangina, hand, mouth, foot disease. There is no prevention or treatment for this virus, but few treatment options can help to reduce the symptoms.

**Crabs:** There is other name for these crabs as pediculosis pubis and these are nothing, but lice within the pubic hair. These lice may be seen present within beard and eyelashes, eyebrows, armpits and chest hair too. There is a huge chance for crabs through sexual contact from the partner and through sharing bed with others. Itching is the primary symptom associated with this infection. These pubic lice can be prevented and eliminated like all other lice.

**Croup:** Croup is an inflammation and air passage narrowing, which can result into wheezing and bark kind cough. It is very commonly seen in children. This is not a serious illness. This croup is caused through many varieties viral infections that are capable enough to affect larynx, airway of lungs and windpipe. This croup generally appear like cold for one to week days and later will turn into fever along with cough and breathing issues. Generally, doctors will identify this croup through the symptoms. Mist vaporizer is a better treatment for this problem. If this croup is not treated, then it can transform into severe complication as tracheobronchitis.

**Cryptococcosis:** This is a rare fungal infection develops through cryptococcus neoformans inhaling. This fungus is commonly seen all over the world. The progressive stage of this infection can be fatal for the victim. Symptoms will mainly dependent over the organ associated with this infection and fever is commonly associated with this infection. For example infected lungs will show symptoms of coughing. This can be diagnosed through identifying the fungi in sputum specimen, spinal fluid, and pus or through tissue biopsy. The choicest drug to treat this issue is Fluconazole.

**Cryptococcus:** This is a yeasty fungus genus and commonly seen in soil. This fungus also can be seen in mucous membranes and over skin of the healthy humans too.

**Cryptosporidiosis:** this is food poisoning protozoan known as cryptospordium. This parasite used to live within the human intestine cells and produces worms. These worms can survive outside the body for a longer duration successfully. This kind of survival buys them thorough entry into the food or water to result into food poisoning. Water diarrhea is the major symptom associated with this infection. This infection can be diagnosed through stool examination. There is no specific treatment for this infection, but some patients will have chance to find some good relief with antibiotics.

**Cryptosporidium:** this is a parasite to cause waterborne infection. Water diarrhea is the result through this infection for a healthy individual. Boiling water can kill these bacteria successfully within a minute. This bacterium is capable enough to survive within chlorine water too.

**Cutaneous Larva Migrans:** This infection is widely popular as creeping eruption and it is caused through Hookworm larvae that normally present within pets and other animals. This Hookworm will attack human skin, when it touches contaminated soil that is with cat or dog feces. Skin lesions are the major symptom for this disease. Generally, hands and feet are more prone to this disease through direct contact with the contaminated soil. The best treatment for this infection is Thiabendazole and applied over the skin tracks and over normal skin.

**Cyclospora cayetanensis:** This is another parasite microbe to infect human intestine to result into diarrhea, fatigue and weight loss. This parasite is still a new organism for scientists as this was appeared very recently. This is distant cousin organism for Crytospordium. Severe diarrhea will start appear within a week duration of ingestion along with cramps, stomachache, vomiting and nausea. Antibiotic combination with trimethoprim and sulfa can help well to shorten the illness of the victim. Here, it is highly imperative to mention that most of the diarrhea causing organisms is nowadays quite resistant with drugs.

**Cytomegalovirus (CMV) Infection:** this infection caused through Herpes virus family and this CMV is a pretty complex virus. This infection can result into problems for pregnancy for a woman that is with acute infection. This CMV is commonly present in human body fluids like urine, semen, saliva, blood, breast milk and some more. It can be transmitted quite easily through sexual intercourse. The symptoms are always mild with this infection with achiness along with low fever and sore throat. Blood test is ideal to confirm CMV. There is no specific cure for CMV and babies should be hospitalized, when attacked by this disease.

# Infectious Diseases Start with "D"

**Dacryocystitis:** This is an inflammation to tear gland or lacrimal sac over corner portion of the eye and this will be caused through duct obstruction. Discharge is a chance through this infection for the eye besides tearing. The acute infection can result into pain and inflammation to sac. This will happen in general to one side and commonly seen with infants. Treatment for this problem is antibiotics with systemic treatment. Very rare cases will demand surgery to keep the duct open through inserting a plastic tube.

**Deet (Diethyltoluamide):** This is one type of insect repellent to be sprayed over the skin to keep away from the disease causing gnats, mosquitoes and similar insects. This is nontoxic, when considered through low level of concentration, but not suitable for children.

**Dengue Fever:** This is another dangerous infectious viral fever comes in four distinct varieties. It will cause rashes and severe joint pains for the victim. This disease generally transmitted through mosquitoes. There is a chance for this fever to turn into dangerous dengue hemorrhagic disease too. This fever is caused through urban aedes mosquito and this mosquito will bite humans during day time indoors. This is termed to be bad flu case through sudden fever. The symptoms can be seen as muscle ache, frontal headache, vomiting, nausea, rashes for 3 to 5 days. It may spread to legs, face, arms and torso down the line. Specific treatment is not available for dengue fever, but painkillers can offer reasonable relief for symptoms.

**Dengue Hemorrhagic Fever Shock Syndrome (DHFS):** This is a grave condition of dengue fever with more chances for hemorrhage and collapse. The cause for DHFS is still not certain, but patient age, immune status and genetic status are the major factors to determine the cause. The symptoms are cold, respiratory distress, thready pulse, weakness and all dengue fever symptoms in addition. Fluid along with electrolyte replacement is the essential treatment for this disease. There is a chance for the requirement of transfusions for blood, platelets and plasma. Sedatives and oxygen support should be provided adequately for the patient.

**Dermatophytes:** This is a superficial fungi also known as tineal infection or ringworm. This disease normally infects hair, skin and nails. The microsporum fungi are the reason for this disease along with trichophyton and epidermophyton.

**Dermatophytosis:** This is another fungus infection caused through trichophyton or through microsporum or through dermophyton.

**Desert fever:** This is widely popular as Coccidioidomycosis.

**Desert Rheumatism:** This is also called as Coccioidomycosis.

**Diarrhea and Infectious Disease:** Many types of infectious diseases can result into diarrhea in humans and watery loose tools on frequent intervals will happen through this disease. Acute diarrhea is a common disease that will happen to most of the humans and this will happen through the consumption of contaminated food. This will start and stays from three hours to three days. This diarrhea will result into loss of fluids within the victim body and treatment will be to replace these fluids along with electrolytes. Very common treatment for diarrhea is to drink water with sugar and salt frequently.

**Diphtheria:** This is a common curable bacterial disease, which tends to affect tonsils, nose, throat or the human skin. This diphtheria is caused through the bacteria known as Corynebacterium diphtheriae. This bacterium survives in dark and wet areas. Mouth, nose and throat are the suitable places for this bacterium to nest within human body. Untreated patient can result into more contagious. This contagious stage will be only up to two weeks after the infection started. The symptoms will begin within five days. There are two varieties of diphtheria as one can affect nose and throat, while the second one can affect skin. This disease is completely preventable and treatable. Diphtheria antitoxin through hospitalization can offer good treatment for this disease.

**Diphtheria, Skin:** This skin diphtheria is generally caused through corynebacterium diphtheriae, which is also reason for the diphtheria in nose and throat. This is a superficial ulcer infection for the skin. Initially, brow-gray or gray-yellow rashes will appear and peel off to turn into brown-black rashes that surrounded with inflammation. There is a chance for nasal discharge too through this disease. The mild cases can be easily treated with antibiotics and antitoxins like Pencillin and V Potassium. Here, antitoxin will result into a great help to inactive the toxin.

**Diphtheria Toxoid:** It is a vaccine to diphtheria produced through combining tetanus toxoid vaccine and pertussis in the injections form. It should be administered while infancy or childhood. Also, you can prepare the same through adding diphtheria toxoid with tetanus toxoid and give it to children. You can add tetanus toxoid to this mixture while treating adults.

**Diphyllobothriasis:** This is a disease caused through the fish tapeworm and this will happen, when eaten infected fish. These are pure parasitic flatworms known as diphyllobothrium latum. The symptoms are distended abdomen, cramping, flatulence, and diarrhea. This infection will show its impact within ten days after eating the infected fish. This disease is generally identified, when found eggs within the feces of the patient. Treatment for this disease is through niclosamode drug from a physician.

**Diphyllobothrium spp:** This is a flattapeworm to cause diphyllobothriasis.

**Disinfectant:** This is a popular chemical germicide for disinfecting the surfaces. It is not suitable for human skin. Most of these disinfectant used in home will contain isopropyl alcohol, ethyl alcohol, ammonia, pine oil, phosphoric acid and hydrogen peroxide.

**Disinfection:** This is used to eliminate germs from the surfaces. Hospitals will generally use low-level disinfectants. The most commonly seen disinfectants are chlorine bleach, chemical disinfectants and alcohol.

**Division of Bacterial and Mycotic Disease:** This is a special division in the U.S.A. for disease control and prevention. This division will extend its services towards the bacteria causing diseases prevention and control.

**Dracunculiasis (Dracontiasis):** This is a disease caused through parasite and affects the humans. This is also known as guinea worm disease too. People will turn into prey for this disease through drinking contaminated water. The worm larvae are capable enough to penetrate into the intestine wall of humans. It will gain entry from there into the skin beneath layer. Here, adult worm will lay embryos through skin opening. This entire process will take approximately thirteen months after drinking the contaminated water. The symptoms are itchy feeling after the worm reaches the skin surface and this will be followed by blisters over the foot or leg of the infected human. There is chance for nausea, vomiting, general itching and fever too. Antibiotics are the good treatment for this problem.

**Dysentery:** This is an infection to result into severe diarrhea. The protozoan Entamoeba hystolytica will cause amebic dysentery. This will transform into intestine ulcer, abscesses in liver, brain, heart and testes slowly. This dysentery is generally caused through genus shigella bacteria, which is contagious through contact or via contaminated water and food.

## Infectious Diseases Start with "E"

**Ear Infection:** The common name of ear infection is Otitis media and this infection involves era's middle portion. This infection will result into pus and severe ache. Very often this infection can result into hear loss too. There are no long-term complications with this infection as it can be treated quite easily. The very common reason for the ear infection is through blocked Eustachian tube, which happens during cold through fluid accumulation in the middle portion of the ear. Acute infection symptoms are severe aching, ringing in the ear, deafness, fullness sense and fever. Chronic infection symptoms are seeping pus and this debris can erode bone too. Diagnosis of this infection will be carried out through Otoscope tool. Antibiotics can clear and clean the acute infection successfully. If this is a persistent infection, then doctor interference is necessary.

**Ebola (hemorrhagic Fever):** This is a deadly illness caused through the Ebola viruses. There are four varieties of Ebola viruses called as filo viruses basing on their appearance. Contaminated blood, feces, vomit and urine can transmit this infection successfully. There is a chance for this virus to attack healthy human, when touched a dead body that is died through Ebola virus infection. Breathing of Ebola virus droplets within the atmosphere also can infect humans. This Ebola hemorrhagic fever symptoms are weakness, headache, muscle pain and throat ache. There is a chance for added symptoms like diarrhea, vomiting, rash, liver failure, abdominal ache, and kidney problems. Blood specimen is essential to diagnosis this infection. Specific treatment is currently not available for this infection and severe cases will deserve hospitalization.

**Echinococcosis:** This is tapeworm infection caused through larvae of the worm, which is called as echinococcus granulosus. Infected pets will transmit this infection to humans and sometimes it will transmit through soil, contaminated water, vegetables and feces of animals too. There will not be any symptoms during early stage of the infection, but after few years cysts will develop in liver of the victim. The possible symptoms after the cysts development will be discomfort abdomen, vomiting, nausea, fever, pain and sometimes can lead to death too. It is tough to diagnosis this infection as early stage will be with no symptoms. The cysts development only can be identified through X-ray or other medical tests. The treatment for this disease is removal of cysts through surgery. Also, taking albendazole and mebendazole can kill the organisms inside the cysts too.

**ECHOvirus:** This is known as Enteric Cytopathogenic Human Orphan that is ECHOvirus. This is a picornavirus with few syndromes. There are more than 30 varieties ECHOviruses were identified so far by scientists. These will cause nonbacterial meningitis.

**Ecthyma:** This is a ulcer kind skin infection results scarring over the skin. This will be almost like Impetigo and develops over legs and other protected portions of the human body. This will be started with single lesion that will grow into big and encrusts. This crust is generally a pus-filled ulcer with lack of hygiene. Antibiotics are the perfect treatment for this infection.

**Ectoparasite:** This parasite lives over the skin for obtaining nourishment through sucking blood of the host. Lice, ticks and some more will also come under this category.

**Ectothrix:** This is a fungus grows hair shaft outside.

**Eczema, Hypeticum:** This is a very rare skin infection happens through Herpes Simplex virus. This will result into extensive blisters and rashes for the victim. Hospitalization is essential to treat this infection and this disease also known as Kaposi's varicelliform eruption too.

**Ehrlichia:** This is a bacterium to infect domestic animals. This bacterium belongs to the Rickettsia family to cause tick-borne disease for humans.

**Ehrlichiosis, Canine:** This disease will happen through Enrlichia bacteria and carried via brown dog tick. This is a dog disease.

**Ehrlichiosis, Equine:** This is a horse disease caused through Ehrlichia equi bacteria.

**Ehrlichiosis, Human Granulocytic:** This disease is generally spread through a tick that is famous for carrying Lyme disease too. Diagnosis of this disease is difficult as there is no standardized testing yet for this disease. The bacteria will start to multiply within ten days after the tick bite in humans. These bacteria will reside within white cells and result into fever. Other symptoms added to fever will be headache, muscle pain, chills, and some more. Prompt and quck treatment is essential for this disease. Delayed cases will be hard to treat. This will respond suitably with doxycycline and tetracycline antibiotics.

**Ehrlichiosis, Human Monocytic:** This disease is generally caused through Ehrlichia Chaffeensis bacteria and these bacteria will be carried normally by the Lone Star tick. This Lone Star tick bite can result into this disease for humans. The symptoms are fever, malaise, chills, sweating, vomiting, nausea, and muscle ache. This can be mild to threatening to result into life threatening disease. Antibiotics are the proven treatment procedure for this disease.

**Elephantiasis:** This is a disease to lead into leg massive swelling through an obstructed lymph vessel. This is caused through the worms' infection and legs are the most affected part of the human body through this disease. There is chance for arms, scrotum or vulva or breast may affect through this disease too. Treatment is not available to reverse the elephantiasis, but enlarged scrotum can be retrieved well through surgery.

**Encephalitis:** This is a viral infection to result into inflammation for brain. The membranes that are covering brain will have more chances to affect through this disease. The responsible virus for this disease are Herpes Simplex virus Type I. The symptoms will be started with headache, prostration and fever. There is a chance for additional symptoms like hallucination, paralysis, confusion, behavioral disturbance, speech problem, and memory problem and eye issues. There is an antiviral drug named as acyclovir, which is to be administered intravenously for the victim. It is an effective treatment option for this disease.

**Encephalitis, California:** This disease will happen through an infected mosquito bite to humans and virus will enter into the bloodstream of human after the bite to reach spine and brain. The virus will start to multiply within the central nervous system of the human to damage nerve cells, inflaming and send s signals to other parts of the body. The symptoms will start with fever along with irritability, headache, vomiting, nausea, drowsiness, seizures and convulsions. This disease diagnosis is possible through lumbar picture. There is no specific cure for this disease and immune system of the victim should always be capable enough to destroy virus.

**Encephalitis, Eastern Equine (EEE):** This is another common arboviral infection and a deadly one too. Four varieties of mosquitoes in general will carry this virus causes EE for humans through their bite. Virus will reach brain and spine after the mosquito bite. Symptoms will begin within 15 days as fever headache, chills, nausea and muscle ache. There is a possibility for coma or paralysis or convulsions through disease for a victim. Rapid test to cerebrospinal fluid and blood should be conducted to diagnosis this disease. There is no specific treatment, but pain killers can help to relive symptoms.

**Encephalitis, Japanese:** This is a zoonosis disease caused through mosquito bite. Culex mosquito will transmit the disease through bite to humans. These mosquitoes will be seen more during fall and summer. The virus will enter into bloodstream and to brain after the mosquito bite. There will be mild symptoms and some will experience no symptoms too. The infection will be active after 8 days to the bite and results into flu kind illness along with headache, stomach issues, fever, behavior problems, confusion and some more. This can lead to paralysis and bran damage too. Rapid test can reveal the disease presence for the victim. There is no treatment for this disease, but symptoms can relieved successfully through hospitalization or medicines.

**Encephalitis Lethargica:** This disease belongs to the encephalitis with symptoms as similar to the Encephalitis along with extreme lethargy and drowsy condition.

**Encephalitis, St. Louis:** This is another arboviral infection affects brain and generally transmitted through birds and infected mosquitoes' bite. The virus enters bloodstream and from there reaches the brain and spine to develop into multiples. The symptoms with disease are flu kind illness along with headache, fever, malaise, stiff neck, convulsions and delirium. The brain CT scan or EEG from doctor can be a right diagnosis for this disease. There is no vaccination or cure for this disease.

**Encephalitis, tick-borne:** This is a viral infection for the human central nervous system through tick bite. Some of the unpasteurized dairy products can also bring this disease to humans. The treatment for this disease is symptomatic.

**Encephalomyelitis:** This is also known as equine encephalitis too. This will cause inflammation for brain of the victim and to spine. Mental impairment is the major symptom associated with this disease along with weakness, discomfort, drowsiness, nausea, headache, confusion, seizures and stiff neck. Specific treatment is not available for this problem.

**Endothrix:** It is superficial fungus resides within hair shaft to grow and to produce spore in a way not to come out of hair.

**Entamoeba Histolytica:** this is a special form of amoeba to cause amoeba dysentery and hepatic amebiasis for humans.

**Enteritis:** this is viral and bacterial infection to cause inflammation for the lining of intestine. If the problem develops with small and large intestines, then this will be termed as enterocolitis.

**Enterobiasis:** this is a parasitic infection for the human intestine through pinworm known as Entrobius vermicularis. This worm generally will infect large intestine and female worms will lay eggs in perianal location. There is a chance for reinfection, when these eggs reached to mouth. Sleeplessness and itchiness are the symptoms associated with this infection. Perianal area should be inspected through applying tape for the worm eggs presence with the help of microscope as a part of diagnosis. The entire family will need treatment, when a family member infected. It is essential for this treatment to destroy all the pinworms as there is a chance for reinfection.

**Enterococcus:** This infection will inhabit gastrointestinal tract of the human. These bacteria are highly resistant with antibiotics.

**Enterobius Vermicularis:** This is a common parasite nematode and a pinworm too.

**Enterotoxin:** This is a poisonous toxin produced by bacteria to create inflammation to intestine lining of the human. This will result into diarrhea and vomiting for the victim. Generally, food will be contaminated trough the enterotoxin that is produced by staphylococci bacteria. Cooking cannot destroy this toxin and it is resistant with heat too.

**Enterovirus:** This is a group virus tries multiply within the intestinal tract of the human. There will be a chance to experience few symptoms for the people that are with these enterovirus. This virus is hard to kill and resistant with antibiotics too. They can survive in temperatures up to 122 degrees F.

**Epidemic:** This is a phenomenon for a disease that will come and transmit all over within a short span of time.

**Epidemiology:** This is a science that handles the determination process for the cause of a disease. This process will include the determination of prevention acts against the disease too.

**Epiglottitis:** This disease is caused through Haemophilus influenzae Type B bacteria. The severe condition of disease can show symptoms as sore throat, noisy breathing, fever, swollen epiglottis and croupy cough. Rest along with antibiotics, supportive care and oxygen are the best treatment procedure for this disease.

**Epstein-Barr virus (EBV):** This is most common universal human virus and causes infectious disease Mononucleosis. This virus belongs to the Herpes family too. This infectious disease generally attacks children below 6 years old. The transmission of EBV is still a mystery, but believed to be causing through infected saliva. This virus will not transmit through blood or air.

**Equine Morbillivirus (EM):** This is a rare infectious disease caused through morbillivirus. Scientists are still clueless about the virus entry and its reappearance. This virus is virulent and 70% cases will experience death through this disease. There is no specific treatment for this disease.

**Erysipelas:** This is a contagious infection caused through streptococcus pyogenes bacteria at skin and its tissues. These bacteria gain entry into the skin through lesions. Sudden fever will start within 7 days after the infection initiated in the body. There will be headache, vomiting and malaise too. Pencillin is the right treatment for this disease. It takes seven days to cure.

**Erythema Annulare Centrifugam:** This is an infection with ring shape plaques. This is a short term problem and happens to all age group individuals. This is caused through Dermatophyte fungus and results into parasitic bowels disease, or cancer or blue cheese ingestion or autoimmune disorder. Regular fungus treating antibiotics can treat this problem effectively.

**Erythema Chronicum Migrans:** This is a skin problem seen in the form of lesions as the first sign. It will start as small and spreads fast.

**Erythema Nodosum:** This is another inflammator skin disease through an infection agent or through drug sensitivity or through Pencillin salicylates. This will happen through streptococcal throat infection and associated with Tuberculosis too. This will start as tender and shiny swelling in 4-inches size over thighs or arms. Fever also is seen with this infection along with muscle pain and joints pain. The treatment for this problem is bed rest along with few suitable painkillers.

**Erythrasma:** this is another bacterial infection with mild itching and burning. This will cause through Corynebacterium minutissimmumSevere cases of this infection can be treated effectively with erythromycin. Ointments like Whitefield and tolnatate can also offer significant good results.

**Escherichia:** This is a gram-negative bacteria present within animal and human intestines.

**Escherichia Coli (E. coli):** This is a coliform bacteria species family and seen in soil, water, intestines and milk. This E.coli is seen in five different groups with toxins that can cause Traveler's Diarrhea.

**Exogenous Infection:** This is an infection develops due to some type of bacteria that is commonly seen outside of the body. These bacteria will not belong to the bacteria population that lives within human.

**Eye Infection:** The common eye infection is known as Conjunctivitis or pink eye. The common reason for eye infection is staphylococci bacteria or through the virus that are associated with sore throat, cold or other illness.

## Infectious Diseases Start with "F'

**Fasciola Hepatica:** This is a liver fluke to cause Fascioliasis.

**Fascioliasis:** This is an infection to liver fluke. This disease is generally caused through Fasciola hepatica virus. The symptoms of this disease are epigastric pain, jaundice, fever, diarrhea and hives. Oral bithionol will be the ideal treatment for this disease.

**Fever:** fever is an abnormal temperature condition for the human body due to a disease. Antipyretics can lower this temperature and results into a good treatment too. Also, aspirin or acetaminophen can be a wise choice for treating fever too.

**Fifth Disease:** This is a viral infection and affects red cells of the blood. This is also known as slapped cheeks too. This disease is generally caused through pavovirus B19. This infection starts with headache in children along with tiredness, muscle pain and rosy red rashes within three days period. Adults will experience fever through this infection along with joint pains similar to arthritis. This disease is often diagnosed through appearance and symptoms. Specific treatment is not available for this disease, but bed rest along with clear fluids and acetaminophen to lower temperature can bring good relief for the victim.

**Filariasis:** This is a tropical disease caused through parasitic roundworms and their larvae. Generally, this infection transmitted to humans through infected mosquito and the larvae will gain entry into the human lymph system with the help of this infected mosquito bite. The symptoms will appear between 3 months and 12 months period with inflammation. This will add up with chills, fever and headache. Blood specimen should be examined for this disease diagnosis. This disease will be easy to treat in the early or mild stage. It is suggested taking three weeks course of diethylcarbamazine.

**Fish and Infectious Disease:** Fish contamination is highly dangerous and bacteria within the fish can result into a great threat for health. Fish often available in the form of frozen and this is tough to judge their status. It is always good to consider fish that is fresh through looks and smell. Its skin and eyes can inform the freshness to a good extent. Fishy smell or ammonia odor fish should be avoided from consumption. Always seek the fish from the bottom area of the freezer. It is always a good idea to scrape fatty skin of the fish before cooking and this can safeguard the contamination to a good extent.

**Flatworms:** There are important two varieties of flatworms that can affect human health and those are cestodes and trematodes.

**Fleas:** Flea bite is most dangerous for humans, which can cause into dangerous disease. These are pure blood suckers and these insects are capable enough to transmit Arboviruses into humans successfully.

**Flesh-Eating Bacteria:** this is a disease, where bacteria releases toxin that enters into the skin to destroys muscles and fat of the victim. Also, this toxin is capable enough to trick the human immune system too. So, this will help well to toxin to improve their attack over fat and muscles. There will be breathing problems with this disease along with symptoms as leg or arm swelling, painful skin, and hot. There is a chance to appear blisters that are with clear fluids. Blood culture can reveal this infection during the diagnosis procedure. Medical attention is necessary to treat this infection. Choicest drug is Pencillin for this disease. It is required to remove infected limb or tissue through surgery.

**Flies and Infections:** Flies are almost like mosquitoes to transmit some types of diseases. Here are more than 65 varieties diseases that are transmitted generally through flies into humans.

**Fluke:** This is a parasite and flatworm belongs to the Trematoda class.

**Folliculitis:** This infection causes to hair follicle through staphylococcus bacteria and chances to appear any part of the skin. Bearded areas are commonly seen with this infection. Antibiotics can treat this problem more effectively.

**Fomites:** These are pure nonliving material like bed linen and transmit diseases and disease causing organism successfully.

**Food Poisoning:** Food poisoning is form of food-borne infection through a toxic process. Contaminated food is the major reason for this problem. This food contamination generally happens through toxic substances or through bacteria or through bacteria hat is containing toxins.

**Fort Bragg Fever:** This is also known as Leptospirosis infection causes through leptospira genus.

**Francisella Tularensis:** This is an infectious disease caused through Tularemia bacteria. This disease can be seen in humans as well as in animals too.

**Fungal Infection:** This is a skin disease caused through fungi. This is harmless fungi and commonly present within the human skin. Immunity system and bacterial competition will not let these bacteria to multiply. This fungal disease is common infection and doctors consider three classes' drugs to fight against this fungal infection.

**Fungi:** Fungi are phylum of plants, which includes rusts, yeasts, smuts, molds, mushrooms and some more.

**Furuncle:** This is also called as Boil too. This is a skin infection from bacteria that gains entry through hair follicle. This will form into a painful pus-filled nodule. This boil generally happens through staphylococcus bacteria, which is more active in skin gland or in hair follicle. The symptoms are redness, pain, and swelling. The treatment for this infection is ideal through local care, incision & drainage, and moist heat.

## Infectious Diseases Start with "G"

**Gangrene:** This is a skin disease in the form of dry gangrene and wet gangrene. Dry gangrene skin will die due to the blood supply blockage without bacterial infection. This is not transmitted to other areas of the skin. This dry gangrene will cause due to arteriosclerosis or through diabetes mellitus. Wet gangrene will happen through bacterial infection of dry gangrene or due to the blood flow blockage after the wound. Wet gangrene will have offensive odor and spreads more rapidly. There is another gas gangrene and this is pure virulent form to the wet gangrene happens through clostridium bacteria. The dry skin area will turn into numb and painful through this infection and eventually tissue dies too. Wet gangrene can be identified through special symptoms such as noxious odor, redness, oozing and swelling. Gas gangrene will have pain, swelling, along with tenderness for wound location. Surgical debridement is essential to treat all types of gangrene. It is a good decision to remove dead tissue before healing process will be initiated too.

**Gas Bacillus:** This gas bacillus will produce gas like byproduct for metabolism like some other bacteria as E. coli and few other clostridia species.

**Gastroenteritis bacterial:** This is a bacterial infection to result into stomach inflammation and intestines inflammation. This gastroenteritis will cause due to Enterotoxins of bacteria. Fever is the major symptom for this disease besides nausea, headache, sickness and diarrhea. This disease will have chance to be mistaken as flu too. Mild cases are easy to treat at home, but chronic conditions will require hospitalization.

**Gastroenteritis, Viral:** This is a viral infection caused through bacteria and symptoms will be lack of appetite, vomiting, violent onset and nausea. Bed rest is ideal treatment for this viral infection and sedation and IV fluids can add up well to the bed rest to recover fast.

**Germ:** Microorganisms are termed as germ and these microorganisms are diseasing causing bacteria. Germ is always a better example for bacterium or virus.

**German measles:** This is also known as Rubella too and it is a viral infection. This viral infection caused through rubella virus. This virus generally transmitted through air from an infected person's coughing or sneezing. Contaminated objects also can transmit this disease successfully to others. Youngsters between 6 to 12 years age are more prone to this disease. This infection initially starts with rash on face and this will spread downwards via arms and legs. Blood test is a common practice to reveal rubella. Specific treatment is still not available for rubella, but acetaminophen can help well to reduce fever and other symptoms to a good extent.

**Germicide:** It is drug generally derived to kill microorganisms.

**Giardia Lamblia:** It is type of protozoa to cause into foul smell.

**Giardiasis:** This is another water-borne infection for intestines. This disease normally spreads through contaminated food or through contaminated water or through hand-to-mouth personal contact. Symptoms will be explosive diarrhea, greasy feces, foul-smell, gas, stomach ache, nausea, loss of appetite, and vomiting. Three stool samples examination is required to confirm the giardiasis in a victim. Generally, acute infection will clears up on own, but antibiotics can quicken the healing process to a good extent. There are medications available for this infection as paromomycin, metronidazole and furazolidone.

**Glanders:** This is another dangerous epidemic infection affects donkeys and horses. Occasionally, this infection is seen in humans too. This infection is a result through the pseudomonas mallei bacteria and this is normally transmitted into humans via horses. Some other domestic animals too can transmit this disease to humans too. This infection will cause ulcer or sometimes into abscess through entering via existing wounds. Early antibiotic treatment is essential for this infection.

**Gonorrhea:** This is a very commonly seen STD cause through Neisseria Gonorrhoeae bacteria. These bacteria will pass into other person during sexual intercourse. Symptoms will begin to appear within three days after the infection transmitted. The common symptoms will happen at genital areas or in throat. There will be pain during urination, urge for frequent urination, white or yellow pus via penis are the common symptoms to prove the gonorrhea presence. Culture of organism from the infected person body fluid will be the right diagnosis for this disease. Pencillin has been a proven treatment for many years for this disease.

**Gonyaulax Catanella:** This is a plankton protozoon to produce toxin ingested through shellfish. Toxic shellfish eating is the major reason for this problem, which tends to Shell fish poisoning. There is a no proven antidote for this poisoning and administering prostigmine can result into effective along with artificial respiration.

**Granuloma:** This is grouping of cells that are associated well with chronic inflammation. This inflammation can happen to any area of the body. There are proofs that leprosy and syphilis to turn into infective granulomas within different organs of the infected individual's body. Here, pyogenic granuloma can be a common and benign skin tumor from a minor injury too. Surgical removal is essential for pyogenic granulomas.

**Granuloma, Infectious:** This is a lumpy lesion granuloma tissue that can transform into a disease like syphilis, tuberculosis or actinomycosis or leprosy. Very often, it may transform into tissue-invading organism too.

**Granuloma Inguinale:** This is a chronic bacterial infection for the human genital area. This is assumed as one of the STDs. This disease will cause through calymmatobacterium granulomatis, which is a tiny gram-negative bacillus. Symptoms will appear between 8 and 80 days after infection. Blisters or lumps will form in the genital area due to this disease. Microscopic examination is vital from the smear taken from lesion to confirm the disease. There are many antibiotics available to treat this disease like streptomycin.

**Gulf war Syndrome, Bacterial Cause:** This is a syndrome identified through its symptoms as muscle pain, joint pain, depression, memory loss, chronic fatigue and skin rashes. This may happen due to chemical weapon exposure or through interaction between vaccines and medications.

**Gum Disease:** Gum disease can be identified through roots infection, bleeding teeth and receding gums. This problem will develop due to the plaque collected over the base of teeth. According to scientists, bacteria settled within the plaque will produce toxin to irritate gums to result into infection, swelling and tenderness. Teeth bleeding are the major symptom with this problem along with reddish and purple color gums and swelling. Oral hygiene is essential treatment for this gum infection. Very often dentists will remove surgically some gum margin for the victims.

**Infectious Diseases Start with "H"**

**Haemophilus:** this is another gram-negative bacterium very commonly seen within the respiratory tract of animals and humans. This genus will have H. influenzae to cause infection to the respiratory tract into a form of meningitis.

**Haemophilus Influenzae Type B (Hib):** This rod type bacterium can result into serious disease especially for children as bacterial meningitis. This bacterium is the major cause for meningitis before vaccination in children. This bacterium can also cause ear infection in children too. This bacteria infected children start witness symptoms within 2 weeks and this meningitis in children may happen suddenly or slowly. Lumbar puncture diagnosis is necessary for this infection from the sample fluid collected from spinal cord. This Hib meningitis can kill children, when not treated with medication. 95% of cases will successfully recover through antibiotics. Children with H. flu meningitis will require hospitalization.

**Hand, Foot and mouth Disease:** This is another infectious disease happens mostly to toddlers. This will result into blisters to palms, mouth inside and soles. This disease is mainly caused through coxsackievirus, which infects through contact via mouth secretions or nose. The symptoms will be seen within 6 days of infection through ulcer in cheeks, gums, or over tongue, along with fever, sore throat, aching, rashes on palms, sole, and fingers and at diaper used places. Tests are needed for exact diagnosis and culture should be collected from stool or lesions. Specific treatment is currently not available for this disease, but painkillers suggested for blisters discomfort relief.

**Hantavirus:** This is a group virus generally carried by mice, rodents, voles and rats. This virus will cause different types diseases like Hantavirus pulmonary syndrome, hemorrhagic fever and some more. This virus will generally transmit to humans through contamination of air from affected rodents and other mentioned creatures. Also, urine and saliva of these affected creatures can also transmit this disease to humans, but it will not transmit from person to person.

**Hantavirus Pulmonary Syndrome:** This is a respiratory illness from Hantavirus to result into gasp for air from the victims through filling the lungs with fluids. This HPS is mainly starts almost like flu kind of illness along with fever, chills, muscle pain, and cough. Most of the cases will be misrecognized this disease as hepatitis too. This virus is capable enough to damage the human kidney and lungs through accumulating fluids, which is most dangerous. There is no specific approved treatment available for this disease yet, but antiviral drug Virazole is going to be a promising invention for this disease from the scientists soon.

**Haverhill Fever:** This disease is generally transmitted to humans by rat bite. The Streptobacillus moniliformis bacteria are reason for this disease. This bacterium is most commonly seen in rat saliva. The symptoms of the disease will start to appear within ten days after the rat bite. The symptoms are fever, vomiting, chills, muscle pain, joint pains, and headache. Lab analysis can diagnosis this disease for humans. There are many antibiotics are available to treat this disease effectively.

**Hearing Loss and Infectious Disease:** Ear infection is common cause for the hearing loss in humans. There are so many bacteria, viruses and parasites to cause into hearing loss for humans besides some of the infectious diseases. Some of the infectious diseases that are possible reasons for the hearing loss are bacterial meningitis, syphilis, borrelia burgdorferi, mycobacterium tuberculosis, cytomegalovirus, measles, mumps, rubella, varicella-zoster, fungal infections, toxoplasma gondii, flukes, and some more.

**Helicobacter Pylori:** This is a stomach ulcer through bacteria and this bacterium is capable enough to survive within stomach though it is full of acids. It will nest safely over the mucous lining of stomach. Symptoms of this stomach ulcer will be nausea, pain, vomiting, and fever and these symptoms will last up to 14 days successfully. This ulcer will turn into chronic gastritis, when not treated. Blood test is right kind of diagnosis for this disease. Combination of antibiotics and anti-ulcer medicines can bring quick relief from the disease.

**Helmimthiasis:** This is an infestation caused through parasitic worm.

**Hemolytic Uremic Syndrome (HUS):** This is one of the rare forms of kidney disease. This is another food-borne disease through escherichia coli bacteria. These bacteria will cause red blood cells damage and bleeding for kidneys. The victim will turn into pale and more tired along with fever and increased blood pressure through this disease. This is a dangerous and life threatening disease deserves hospitalization and intensive acre without fail.

**Hepatitis:** This is a disease to cause inflammation to liver and this is generally caused through virus. In some cases this hepatitis can happen due to alcohol or through usage of certain drugs that leads into liver damage. Liver function will be totally inappropriate through hepatitis. Jaundice is the sign of the liver wrong functioning and deserves hospitalization. Severe hepatitis case will lead to death or else requiring liver transplant.

**Hepatitis A:** this is a low danger hepatitis cause through virus. This is a food-borne virus successful to replicate within liver. This Hepatitis A will cause through contaminated food and water consumption, which contains terovirus group in it. Hepatitis A will hardly have any symptoms, but children will tend to have mild symptoms. Blood test is vital diagnosis procedure to find out this disease. There is no specific treatment, but patients are suggested having rest and healthy diet.

**Hepatitis B:** this is initially named as serum hepatitis and its quite preventable disease too. This Hepatitis B causes through hepatitis b virus and this is transmitted similar way like in AIDS virus. This disease will not spread through contact. Virus needs to enter into the blood to infect. Symptoms of Hepatitis B will take up to 6 weeks duration to show impact. The symptoms are nausea, tiredness, muscle pain, joints pain, and abdominal pain, loss in appetite, rashes, and mild diarrhea. Hepatitis B can be diagnosed through blood test. Chronic Hepatitis B can be treated successfully with alpha-interferon. It is quite imperative to mention that this interferon will have short-term side effects over the users as fever, loss in appetite, chills, sleep problems, vomiting, and some more. Here is no treatment available for acute Hepatitis B and bed rest is reasonably enough.

**Hepatitis C:** This Hepatitis C is blood-borne disease capable to stay within the body quite for many years. This will spread initially through all the possible blood-related sources like transfusions, drug usage, and dialysis of kidneys. The risk of transmission through sex is very nominal with Hepatitis C. It will not transmit through contact too. There is a chance for the infected mother to transmit this disease to the new born. The symptoms are loss with appetite, nausea, fatigue, stomach pain, vomiting, and jaundice. These symptoms will appear between two weeks and six months after the infection. There is specific cure for this disease, but FDA approved recombinant alpha-interferon.

**Hepatitis D:** This is completely uncommon version of hepatitis and so far infected around 15 million humans. Contaminated needles are the major reason for the hepatitis D and it cannot be transmitted through sex too. Symptoms are hard to distinguish from other hepatitis. This can be diagnosed through finding HDV antigen from liver biopsies or through antibodies within the blood. There is still no reliable treatment for this disease.

**Hepatitis E:** This Hepatitis E is almost similar to A and seen in the epidemic and sporadic ways. This Hepatitis E is generally transmitted via fecal-oral route. It is easy to transmit through water or from person to person. Contaminated food is highly possibility for the transmission of this disease. The symptoms will start to appear between two and nine weeks period. The symptoms are malaise, abdominal pain, anorexia, and fever. This disease can be identified through symptoms. Antiviral treatment is not effective for this disease, but ribavirin and alpha-interferon may help up to a good extent.

**Hepatitis F:** This virus is still under scanner and very little information is currently available about this virus.

**Hepatitis G:** This Hepatitis G is community-acquired acute viral infection. This virus can be transmitted successfully through sexual intercourse and through infected blood. This hepatitis is seen highly with homosexual men. This virus stays within infected human with no symptoms for years. According to researches, this virus will replicate within liver to result into damage for liver eventually. Special liver function test is required to diagnosis this Hepatitis G. There is no specific proven treatment for this disease. Also, there is no test available to screen the blood for the presence of Hepatitis G virus too.

**Herpes:** It is a skin disease starts with blister through the herpes simplex virus. This will result into cold sores and genital herpes will result into blisters over sex organ. There two types of virus to cause this disease and those are Herpes Simplex Type 1 and Type 2. Type 1 virus will cause herpes to lips, face and mouth. Type 2 will cause genital herpes. Initial stage of the herpes will have no symptoms and almost looks like flu. Slowly, ulcer will start to appear over skin at areas as mouth and virus stays within face nerve cells. There is a chance for the recurring infection through the virus that is settled within the face nerve cells. Treatment for herpes should be carried out basing on its severity and location over the skin. Currently acyclovir antiviral drug is helping well for the victims and it will reduce the symptoms to a good extent. His should be administered during early stages of the infection for obtaining effective results. Also, prophylactically is another drug that can control future attacks of the infection too.

**Herpes, Genital:** This Herpes Genital is next to AIDS in the list of highly sexually transmitted diseases. This will cause through Herpes Simplex Type 2 virus. This virus is capable enough to attack skin or any other mucous membrane surface of the infected individual body. If an individual with cold sore engaged in oral sex, then herpes can be transmitted to genitals of the sexual partner. This infection can be transmitted through contact through genital secretions of the individual that is with active lesion. 40% of infected people only will experience symptoms with this disease as rest will not have any symptoms. Primary lesion would be the worst stage of this infection. Pain in lesions will stay up to ten days. Virus will stay inside though the lesion healed well. Genital herpes only can be diagnosed through symptoms. Acyclovir is ideal antiviral drug for this infection, but it will not kill the virus permanently. It is available in the form of capsules, ointment, IV form and as fluids.

**Herpes Simplex Type 1 (HSV 1):** This is a member of herpes family to cause herpes to face, mouth and lips.

**Herpes Simplex Type 2 (HSV 2):** This is another member of herpes family to cause genital herpes.

**Histoplasma capsulatum:** This is a fungal organism to cause Histoplasmosis. This fungus generally spread through air-borne spores from the contaminated soil that is with bird droppings.

**Histoplasmosis:** This is a disease happens through inhaling fungus spores known as histoplasma capsulatum. Soil will be contaminated through chicken, pigeon and some other birds' infected excreta and this will mix up with the atmosphere along with spore of fungus. A person that is inhaled these spores will be attacked by this disease. There will be no symptoms during initial stage with this disease. Symptoms down the line would be with breathlessness, joint pain, cough, and some more. Usually, there will be spontaneous recovery, but little calcification will stay in lymph glands and lungs. Tissue or sputum examination is required for the diagnosis. Antifungal toxicities are available to treat this issue effectively. Severe stage should be treated with amophotericin B, which is an effective antifungal drug.

**Hookworm Disease:** This disease will cause through blood-sucking worms. The hookworm larvae generally will be in the soil and gains entry into the human skin to infect. This larvae will reach lungs and into small intestine after gaining entry through skin. These worms will start to suck blood from there successfully. Heavy worm attack can result into severe damage for intestine walls. Minor infection will not show any symptoms, but severe cases will have abdominal pain, diarrhea, anemia, mental inertia, cough, and pneumonia along with itchy rash. Mebendazole is an antihelminthic drug and it is an ideal choice to treat this problem effectively. This drug can kill the worms successfully and requires blood transfusion and healthy diet to recover faster.

**Human Immunodeficiency Virus (HIV):** This is a retrovirus type to cause AIDS. This virus will infect T-helper cells of human immune system and results into slow onset symptoms for the victim. There is a chance for the attack through Kaposi's sarcoma, Tuberculosis, pneumonia candidiasis and pneumocystis carini as the immune system is damaged through HIV. Antibody test is the best diagnosis procedure to find out the HIV in humans.

**Humidifiers and Infectious Diseases:** Winter season will demand the usage of humidifiers, which can help to keep the mucous membranes to be healthy and moist, but poorly maintained humidifiers can result into a best source for the infections. Here, it is a good practice to not let the humidifier function above 40% in order to keep the infection causing molds and bacteria away. It is a good practice to clean the humidifier water reservoir on regular basis with vinegar solution.

# Infectious Diseases Start with "I"

**Immune Response:** Immune response is condition for the body to defend against invading organism that is identified as foreign for the body. This response procedure will trigger antibodies, cells and lymphocytes creation to destroy the invaders successfully.

**Immune System:** There are wide varieties of infections to infect human body and body will try to protect against these invaders through all possible measures. This protection or safeguard procedure by the body will be carried out through combination of cells and organs and this is called immune system. This immune system network will be more effective, when the person having enough rest, less stress and healthy diet.

**Immunity:** This is a quality that indicates protection against the infectious diseases and conditions effectively for the human body.

**Immunization:** This is an artificial method of creating immunity against a disease. Vaccination is the primary option for the immunization. Treated antigens will be arranged through injection in immunization vaccine, which can stimulate produce to create own antibodies for a particular disease successfully. Very often, the contents of the vaccine could be live bacteria, or virus treated in a way to be harmless. Similarly, dead organisms are also used for vaccine to produce the similar effect.

**Immunization for Adults:** Aged individuals that are above 65 years of age require vaccine for various infectious diseases like tetanus diphtheria and some more.

**Immunization for Chronic Disease patients:** Some of the chronic diseases like lung issues, heart problems, diabetes, kidneys problem and sickle cell disease require pneumococcal vaccine and Influenza vaccine during every fall.

**Immunization for Health Care Professionals:** Health care professionals are suggested having several types immunizations, when they come in contact with patients.

**Immunization for Homosexual Mlaes/Heterosexuals with Multiple partners:** It is a great necessary to have Hepatitis B vaccine for the people that are with sexual history.

**Immunization for Institutionalized patients:** It is highly recommended to have Hepatitis B vaccine for the people that are mentally disabled living in institutions.

**Immunization for Kidney Disease patients:** It is recommended to have three doses of Hepatitis B vaccine for the people had kidney transplant and people with hemodialysis.

**Immunization for Patients with Impaired Immune System:** Each fall Influenza vaccine is necessary for the people with impaired immune system.

**Immunization for Pregnant Women:** It is essential for the pregnant women to have live virus vaccines after delivery that are not immune with measles, rubella and mumps.

**Immunization for Public safety Workers:** People that are into public safety field suggested having Hepatitis B vaccine, Influenza vaccine and MMR vaccine without fail.

**Immunization for Research lab workers:** People that are working for research labs and handles specimens that are with poliovirus should have inactivated poliovirus vaccine. Similarly, people that with Plague bacteria research should have plague vaccine. People into Anthrax bacteria research should have anthrax vaccine. People work with Rabies virus should have rabies preventive vaccine.

**Immunization for Veterinarians:** It is highly recommended for veterinarians to have rabies vaccine and blood test for every 2 years.

**Impetigo, Bullous:** his is a superficial skin infection known as staphylococcal impetigo too. This infection caused through staphylococcus aureus bacteria. Symptoms will be thin flaccid bullae that can be ruptured quite easily and it will be with fluid or pus. These lesions will be normally seen as groups in an area and ruptured bullae dries up fast to result into shiny veneer, which will be different than thick crust. Antibiotics are best option to treat bullous impetigo and common impetigo. Tropical treatment will not be of any help for this problem.

**Impetigo, Common:** This is superficial skin infection commonly seen in children. This will happen through streptococcal bacteria. If not treated, then it will spread fast all over. The problem will start with tiny blister over skin and looks like an insect bite. These lesions generally happen over scalp, face, and extremities. Oral antibiotics are the right treatment for this common impetigo.

**Infection Control:** This is a procedure to control community-acquired or hospital-acquired infections from spreading to others.

**Infectious Disease:** Infectious disease is one that is caused through a microorganism. These organisms can be seen in three forms as fungi, virus and bacteria. These organisms will look simple, but multiply quite faster than the expectations. These infectious diseases will cause through damage creation to cell and tissues by the microorganisms and toxins released by them. Human immune system should always be strong enough to fight against these infectious diseases. Treatment for most of the infectious diseases can be concluded with antibiotics and antimicrobial medicines.

**Influenza:** this is more contagious respiratory infection and leads into pneumonia very often. This influenza will cause through Influenza A and Influenza B virus. The symptoms will be fever, body aches, and headache. There is a chance to have sore throat too. Diagnosis for

Influenza is very costly and this is generally identified through symptoms than the costly lab tests. Here, specific treatment is not available for Influenza, but antibiotics will be prescribed to reduce the symptoms and fever.

**Insects and Disease:** There are more than one million species of insects live all around us. Most of these insects are helpful and harmless too. Harmful insects generally will cause infections for humans.

**Interferon:** this is a natural protein developed through infected cells along with virus that is capable enough to interfere with the viral growth.

**Isolation Precautions:** This is a procedure to keep infected patient in an isolated room to keep away from infecting to others.

## Infectious Diseases Start with "J"

**Jarisch-Herxheimer Reaction:** This is reaction normally follows with syphilis treatment. This will happen due to the death of antigens. This reaction will generally come along with headache and fever. It is tough to prevent this reaction while treating syphilis.

**Jock Itch:** This is also known as tinea cruris too and it is fungal infection. This infection generally caused through Trichophyton or epidermophyton or microsporum. These fungi live commonly over skin tissue nails and hair. The symptoms are mild annoying infection along with red itchy scales. These will generally spread from genitals to thighs inside. Fungal culture collected from skin scraping can diagnosis this problem easily. Antifungal drugs are wise choice to treat this problem. Here, lotions or ointments or creams can offer relief from itchy rashes quickly.

**Jungle Fever:** This is also known as Yellow Fever too.

**Infectious Diseases Start with "K"**

**Kaposi's Sarcoma:** This is malignant skin tumor happens to AIDS patients. This disease also can associate with diabetes, some special disorders and malignant lymphoma. Symptoms will be nodules with blue-red to brown. These will start over feet and ankles to slowly spread towards upper leg. Treatment for this disease low-dose radiation for mild cases and severe cases will deserve anticancer drugs.

**Kawasaki Disease:** This is serious and rare disease to happen with infants with rash. It can be seen in children below five years age too. This infection will not appear and transmission from one to other is still uncertain for scientists. High fever is the symptom associated with this infection, which stays for almost five days. It will not respond to antibiotics. Victim will experience swelling to lymph nodes, irritability, red eyes, and some more. Hospitalization is required for this infection to watch the symptoms as antibiotics can't be of any help.

**Kerion:** This is an immune reaction seen in the form of inflammation over skin. This can be identified through red and pustular swelling, which can stay up to a period of two months. There will be scarring and permanent hair loss at the affected area after clearing. Swelling generally clears up on won, but itchthamnol paste can be applied over swelling as antifungal agents for quick relief.

**Kidney Disorders, Infectious:** Kidney infection is known as Pyelonephritis. This will happen due to the obstruction developed in the urine flow within the urinary tract. Stagnation of urine will be the cause for this kidney disorder.

**Kitchen Infections:** Kitchen is the perfect nest for many types of microbes and deadly organisms. Most varieties of bacteria will tend to settle over sink or drain or over kitchen sponge. These microbes and organisms will produce dangerous organic substances for their own survival. There are many types of detergents are available to remove these microbes and microorganisms successfully from the kitchen. It is highly imperative to be precautious towards this deadly virus, microbes and organisms, which can cause many types of infections for the people.

**Klebsiella:** This is a bacterium genus looks like tiny plump rod and causes several types of respiratory diseases for humans.

## Infectious Diseases Start with "L"

**Lassa fever:** This is a novice viral infection happens at tropical regions. This Lassa virus generally found in one type of rodent species, but transmission is not yet identified. This virus will be seen in all types of fluids in a victim body. Diagnosis should be confirmed only Lassa fever test. Isolated treatment is essential for the victim until recovery. There is no specific treatment for this disease, but medication will be offered to reduce the impact of symptoms. The symptoms are high fever along with cough vomiting, and weakness and these symptoms will appear within three weeks after exposure.

**Legionella Pneumophillia:** This legionnaire's disease will cause through gram negative bacteria.

**Legionnaires' disease:** This is a bacterial infection happens in two different varieties. This can be seen as Legionnaires' disease or as Pontiac fever. Here, Legionnaires' disease is severe condition combined with pneumonia and Pontiac fever is milder condition disease. This disease causes through legionella pneumophilla virus. This disease can be transmitted, when took bath in bacteria contained water. The symptoms will happen within ten days after infection. Symptoms are fever, cough and chills. The diagnosis of this disease is very difficult and requires conducting wide varieties tests. The proven treatment for this disease is erythromycin and rifampin also can be a good choice.

**Leishmania:** This is a parasite protozoan and infects humans through sand-flies. These bacteria can cause Leishmaniasis for humans.

**Leishmaniasis:** This is an infection affects mucous membranes and skin. These bacteria can gain entry into the humans through a sand fly bite. The symptoms are fever, weight loss, spleen swelling, and anemia and liver problems. The treatment for this disease mainly dependent over the geographic strains and effective drugs are available to treat all types of Leishmaniasis.

**Leprosy:** This is a chronic infection, which is capable to damage nerves that are within skin, face and limbs. There will be so many complications with the disease, when not treated. Leprosy develops through Mycobacterium Leprae bacteria, which will spread within nasal mucous as droplets. Nerve will be damaged initially through this disease and starts with darkening the skin. Several antibiotic agents are available to treat leprosy effectively. Usage of two to three antibiotics combination can bring good and faster results.

**Leptospirosis:** This is very infectious disease happens through spirochete leptospira interrogans bacterai. This will be transmitted via urine of the domestic or wild animals. Rats and rodents will have more chances to transmit this disease to humans. This disease will occur in two stages. The first stage of the disease will begin after three weeks of infection. Acute illness will be the symptom of the first stage along with headache, chills and fever. The next phase will start as Weil's syndrome within ten days after the fever clears up. Bacteria will start to reach brain in the second stage to result into meningitis. Diagnosis needs testing blood, urine, and fluid from the victim. Erythromycin and tetracycline will be effective against this disease.

**Lice:** This is a wingless insect of sesame seed size and with six legs. These lice feed on human blood and reside within human hair. Lice infestation starts with nits and these nits must be eliminated.

**Listeria Monocytogenes:** This is belongs to bacteria species and capable enough to infect wild and domestic animals. These bacteria will cause meningoencephalitis.

**Listeriosis:** This is a food-borne disease with no symptoms. This disease caused through group of Listeria monocyctogenes bacteria. These bacteria are generally seen in cow milk, human and animal feces, soil, and within leafy vegetables. This will be flu kind illness with no special symptoms to mention in adults. Antibiotics are wise choice to treat this disease in adults, children and in pregnant women.

**Loiasis (Loaisis or Loaiasis):** This disease happens through bite of an African deer fly that is already infected. The larvae will turn into adults within human body and adult worm is capable to live up to 15 years period. It takes several years to show any symptoms after the fly bite. In very rare cases symptoms will appear within 4 months. These migrating worms will cause allergy as calabar swellings to legs and arms. Worm will release some metabolic product to sensitize the victim. This painful swelling will stay for five days, but it is recurrent swellings. The drug called Diethylcarbamazine will be a right choice to treat this problem. This drug also can act as a preventive drug too.

**Lyme disease:** This disease causes through Borrelia Burgdorferi bacteria. These bacteria transmitted into humans through deer tick. There will be one to two symptoms to witness with infected individual. Tiny red spots will appear and expand within few weeks in different shapes over the skin. The redness area found at the bite location will have no itching or pain. Some neurological issues also will develop to the victim. Antibiotics like Tetracycline and amoxicillin will help well to heal this disease well.

**Lymphangitis:** This is an infection caused through streptococci bacteria and transmits through an open wound thru lymphatic channels. Red streaks will appear at the infected area and will extend up to nearest lymph node. There will be fever, headache, chills and general illness. Treatment for this infection will be antibiotics along with moist compress.

**Hymphogranuloma Venereum (LGV):** This is a STD involves lymph glands that are within genital area with strains of specific Chlamydia. This infection generally transmitted through sexual intercourse. Small painless pimples will appear as a first symptom to the disease over penis or vagina. These pimples will arrive within 30 days after infection. Slowly, the infection will spread to groin lymph nodes and to surrounding tissue. Tetracycline is a perfect antibiotic to treat this disease.

## Infectious Diseases Start with "M"

**Mad Cow Disease:** This disease causes from cattle to cattle or cattle to human. Also, some scientists mention that this disease will result through eating brain tissue or spine of the infected cow too. Symptoms will appear between 2 and 8 years of time span and includes nervousness, clumsiness, and brain impairment. There is a no special test available to diagnosis this disease in animals, but dead animal brain tissue testing can reveal the disease presence if any. There is no specific cure for Mad Cow disease and available treatment is pure symptomatic.

**Malaria:** This malaria caused through 4 varieties of species belongs to the Plasmodium parasite. This infection is generally transmitted through Anopheles mosquito bite. Symptoms will start to appear within 12 days after the mosquito bite. Early signs look like flu along with fever, headache, chills, muscle pain and malaise. Malaria can be diagnosed through blood smear test. Malaria will be easy to treat during early stages. Severe stage can turn into dangerous complications. Suitable and effective drugs to treat malaria are quinacrine, chloroguanide and chloroquine.

**Marburg Virus:** This is belongs to the exotic filovirus family with 25% fatality rate. This virus first time identified in the year 1967 in Marburg of Germany and inherited the name.

**Mastitis:** This is an infection to breast happens while breast-feeding. Many doctors identified acute mastitis during first two months nursing. This infection is a result through streptococcal or straphylococcal bacteria. Breast will experience pain through this infection along with redness and swelling near to the lymph nodes. There is a chance to form into abscess, when not treated. The ideal treatment for this infection will be pain killers, antibiotics, rest and warm soaks.

**Mastoiditis:** There is a prominent bone rear side to ear known as mastoid bone. Due to the otitis media these mastoid bone will affect and resulted mastoiditis affects children and chances for hearing loss too. This infection happens, when infection spreads up to middle ear portion in mastoid bone. Severe ear ache is the important symptom for this disease. This will add up with headache, and fatigue. There is a chance for fever, discharge through ears, and progressive hearing loss. Physical examination can reveal the mastoiditis. This infection is tough to treat and requires intravenous antibiotics for too long period. In some cases surgery only can clear this infection.

**Measles:** This disease causes through measles virus that is spread via air from the nasal secretions. Symptoms will come out after 11 days. Infants less than six months of age will rarely infect with this disease. Symptoms will be high fever along with general sickness, red eyes, stuffy nose, cough and some more. Physicians can diagnosis measles through symptoms. Treatment for measles is not available yet, but symptoms should be treated with acetaminophen and fluids. Antibiotics will result into in vain against this virus.

**Meningitis:** This is a viral infection caused through fungi or bacteria or virus to the human membranes that cover the spine and brain. The meningitis happened through bacteria will be more serious than rest. This bacterial meningitis will happen through strptococcus pneumoniae or through haemophilus influenzae. Viral meningitis is less dangerous and rarely turns into fatal. This meningitis characterized through headache, irritability, neck stiffness, vomiting, malaise, and nausea.

**Meningitis, Bacterial:** The common two reasons to happen bacterial meningitis are meningococcal meningitis and pneumococcal meningitis. There are childhood vaccines are available to avoid meningitis and these vaccines almost vanished this disease from happening.

Symptoms are high fever along with chills, stiff neck, vomiting and chronic headache. Cephalosporins are the currently used antibiotic to control bacterial meningitis.

**Menigitis, Meningococcal:** This meningococcal meningitis will happen through neisseria meningitidis bacteria. This infection happens through mouth to mouth contact or through indirect contact too. Mild upper-respiratory problems will develop in the patient through this disease. The symptoms are sudden fever, stiff neck, chills, headache, vomiting and nausea. Pencillin G is the perfect treatment for this disease and administered intravenously. Supportive care is necessary for some patients along with antibiotics.

**Meningitis, Pneumococcal:** this is fatal version meningitis caused through streptococcus pneumoniae. This meningitis will cause ear infection, sinusitis and pneumonia besides meningitis to patients. The symptoms for this disease are high fever, vomiting, chills, headaches, stiff neck and seizure. Lumbar puncture test should be performed to diagnosis this disease in a patient. Some varieties of this pneumonia is completely resistant with Pencillin. Hospitalization along with IV drugs can bring reasonable relief to patients. Painkillers and antibiotics to control fever should be added to the treatment.

**Meningitis, Viral:** This type of meningitis caused through virus and less complicate too. This is a mild illness condition for the infected individual. His disease will cause through enteroviruses and this virus generally transmits through fecal-oral route into the humans. This virus can transmit to others through direct contact or through infected feces or through throat and nose secretions. Symptoms to this disease will appear all of sudden with high fever, headache, vomiting and nausea. This viral meningitis can be diagnosed with the help of lumbar puncture. Viral meningitis has no cure, but immune system of the human will be capable enough to come up with antibodies to destroy total virus. Hospitalization along with IV fluids and painkillers will be good choice, when attacked viral meningitis.

**Meningococcus:** This is a bacterium to cause meningitis in human. These bacteria normally present in nose and throat.

**Meningoencephalitis:** This is a bacterial infection to cause inflammation to meninges and brain.

**Meningoencephalitis, Primary Amebic (PAM):** This is a severe infection caused through free-living single-cell ameba. This ameba generally present in freshwater. This ameba generally stay in soil like a cyst and reactivates, when came in contact with water. This ameba reach healthy individual through nose while swimming or bathing in freshwater that is with ameba. These disease symptoms are fever, vomiting, headache and encephalitis. It will slowly lead to coma too. This disease requires treatment in early stages with the help of amphotericin B.

**Meningomyelitis:** This is an infection to cause inflammation to spine and its surrounded membranes.

**Microban:** This is an antibacterial product from FDA with completely odorless and colorless status. This will result into a protection against the growth of fungus, mold and bacteria. It is completely wash proof and can be kept safely within hospital equipment, toys, and some more suitable items.

**Microbes:** Microbes are a kind of life-forms that are too small and hard to see through naked eye. Some of these microbes are in different sizes and shapes. Few of these are tough to see through microscope too. Many scientists believe that the microbes were the first life-forms on this earth. Microbes play a vital role in the environment. Human body other than brain is full of bacteria. Here, it is quite imperative to mention that the human feces are made of 94% microbes.

**Microsporum:** this is a genus belongs to the dermatophytes family and causes Tinea capitis or ringworm to children.

**Microsporum Canis:** this is fungi and seen very often among pet animals like cats and dogs. It is also seen in humans too and causes ringworm.

**Molluscum Contagiosum:** This is a viral infection completely harmless. This infection will show up tiny white lumps over skin surface of palms, soles and hands. This infection happens through poxivirus as skin disease, but it will be more rampant with AIDS patients. The symptoms are shiny pimples along with central depression. These pimples very often happen at genitals, face and thighs. Direct examination requires to diagnosis this infection. This infection generally clears up in few months with healthy people and no treatment necessary. It is essential to consult doctor, when AIDS patient infected with this disease.

**Monkeypox:** This is a genetic cousin to the popular smallpox virus. This monkeypox happens to monkeys, but chances are there to infect and kill humans too. This disease can transmit from person to person and monkey to person. Rashes similar to smallpox will appear as symptoms to the infection. These rashes will appear all over from head to toe as blisters. There will be high fever along with few respiratory problems. The vaccinia vaccine is derived to protect against the smallpox and this same vaccine will work well for monkeypox too.

**Mononucleosis, Infectious:** it is an acute variety herpesvirus infection develops through epstein-barr virus. This disease will happen through EBV droplets, but not a contagious one. Symptoms will develop after 6 weeks to the infection. Those symptoms are sore throat, swelling to lymph glands, fatigue, and bruises. Symptoms are the only way to diagnosis this infection. Specific treatment is currently not available for this disease and symptom management can be carried out through some of the proven antibiotics.

**Morbidity and Mortality Weekly Report:** This is a weekly epidemiologic report about the occurrence of communicable diseases and deaths. This report will cover 120 urban places all over the U.S.A.

**Mosquito Bites:** Mosquitoes are very commonly seen all over the world. Generally, mosquito bite causes swelling along with itching for few days. Here, it is quite imperative to mention that these bites are often infectious trough transmitting their saliva into humans.

Mosquitoes will spread too many numbers of diseases to humans. There are many eradication measures under research against these disease causing mosquitoes.

**Multiple Sclerosis and Viruses:** This is a chronic disease affects nervous system and happens to all age group humans. There is a chance for this infection to damage the sheaths that are covering nerves within spine and brain too. This disease can damage different areas of spine and brain of the infected human.

**Mumps:** this is an acute viral illness and this is one time disease to happen during childhood. Mumps generally spread through airborne droplets that were came out from the infected individual cough or sneeze. This virus is capable enough to invade parotid gland through multiplication. Symptoms will appear within three weeks after the infection. Those symptoms are mild discomfort at angle of the jaw and few will show no symptoms at all. Mumps can be diagnosed only through symptoms. Painkillers are the only available treatment for mumps as there is no specific treatment yet for this disease.

**Mycetoma:** This is rare and tropical infection to bone and skin. This disease is caused through fungi or through actinomycetes bacteria. Antibiotics are available to treat this disease effectively.

**Mycobactetium:** This is rod-shape bacteria with several species in it and causes leprosy and tuberculosis.

**Mycobacterium Avium Complex (MAC):** These MAC organisms are generally found in water, vapor, mist, dust, soil, and in bird droppings. This virus will gain entry into the human body through contaminated food and through water. There is a chance to inhale the virus from air too. The common symptoms associated with this disease are fever, weight loss, night sweat, appetite loss, progressive diarrhea and fatigue. The available treatment for this disease is TB drugs as MAC bacteria related to the organism that results into TB.

**Mycobacterium Leprae:** This is also known as Hansen's bacillus too. This organism causes into leprosy for humans.

**Mycobacterium Tuberculosis:** This is also called as Koch's bacillus and it is slow growth organism. It is the cause to result into tuberculosis in humans.

**Mycology:** This mycology is about study of fungi and fungoid diseases.

**Mycoplasma:** This is other free living bacteria without cell wall. This mycoplasma pneumonia will cause through M. pneumoniae organism that is related mostly to bacteria. This disease will spread through the droplets from throat and nose of the infected person. This transmission will happen, when infected person sneeze or cough. Symptoms will start after 25 days from the infection. Those are dry cough, sore throat, fever, malaise and headache. This may cause into ear infection in few cases too. Symptoms are only possibility to diagnosis this disease. Erythromycin and tetracycline are the effective antibiotics to treat this disease well.

**Mycotoxicosis:** this is a type of fungus-derived metabolite. This can be seen in certain food and capable to result into food poisoning too.

**Myiasis, Cutaneous:** This is an infection caused through fly larvae infestation. Larvae from egg will successfully gain entry into the skin to cause swelling like a boil. This infestation should be avoided to prevent this disease. Covering your wounds will be the best option to prevent this infestation. Treatment for this problem is through applying oil, which can suffocate swelling caused through larvae. This suffocation will let the virus come out of boil to the surface and remove them properly.

**Myocarditis:** This is an acute disease to result into inflammation to the myocardium, which is heart muscle. This will happen though bacterial or fungus or viral infection. This infection may lead to rheumatic fever too. The main cause to happen myocarditis is through chagas disease parasite. Symptoms will vary basing on the type of infection. Also, inflammation and degree of damage also depends over the type of infection with this disease. The common symptoms are fatigue, fever, pain, and slow heartbeat. There is no treatment required as most of the cases clears up on own within few days. Inflammation can be reduced with the help pf prescribed drug Corticosteroid. It is a good idea to have pain killers and bed rest as a part of the treatment for this disease.

**Myxovirus:** this is medium-size virus causes parainfluenza, mumps and influenza.

# Infectious Diseases Start with "N"

**Nanophyetiasis:** This is an infection causes to humans through a parasitic worm. This infection causes through nanophyetus salmincola or through N. schikhobalwi worm. These symptoms will appear this disease look like diarrhea. There will be significant abdominal discomfort through disease along with nausea. This disease identification normally carried out through finding eggs in the infected individual's feces. Treatment for this disease will be effective with niclosamide or bithionol.

**National Center for Infectious Diseases:** This is a surveillance, prevention, research and training institute of infectious diseases. This NCID is also equipped with a division as Vector-borne infectious diseases too. Here, DVBID also serves as international reference center too for the vector-borne bacterial or viral diseases.

**National Institute of Allergy and Infectious Diseases:** This is a federal research institute to provide support for scientists that are conducting research for the improved diagnosis, treatment and prevention of infectious diseases, allergic diseases and over immunology. This NIAID comprised of four divisions in it as AIDS, Microbiology & Infectious diseases, Allergy, Immunology & Transplantation, and Extramural activities.

**Neisseria Gonorrhoeae:** Tis gonorrhea causes through gram-negative bacteria and widely known as diplococcus or gonococcus. Most of the species belongs to this bacteria are resistant to Pencillin and some species can be treated successfully with tetracycline.

**Nitric Oxide:** This is a simple molecule comprised of oxygen and atom along with nitrogen. This is a great help for the immune system to combat against certain varieties of infections. It is widely known as toxic gas too.

**Nocardiosis:** This is a fungus kind infection happens all over the world. This infection caused through Nocardia asteroides bacteria that belong to aerobic species of actinomycetes. This infection is almost similar to pneumonia and cough and fever will be there to the infected person. Sometimes, this infection will leads to abscesses too. Sulfonamide is right drug for this infection to be used for 18 months and adding some more antibiotics to this drug can bring quick and improved results over the victim.

**Norwalk Agent (Virus) Infection:** This is gastroenteritis viral infections causes through several viruses that belong to Norwalk family. This infection generally transmitted through contaminated food ingestion or through contaminated water. This infection can transmit easily from one to other. Very often, salad ingredients or shellfish kind of food contain these Norwalk family virus to result into this disease. Symptoms will start to appear within three days after the infection. There will be abdominal cramps, vomiting, fatigue, mild diarrhea, and muscle pain. There is a possibility to recover from these mild symptoms within two days. This virus presence can be identified in the lab through stools sample or through blood test. This kind of diarrhea caused through virus has no specific treatment. Very commonly antibodies will develop within the infected person to combat against this virus successfully. Rest along with fluids replacement can help well to recover from tis infection and painkillers can be used to gain relief from symptoms.

**Onchocerciasis:** This is a tropical disease result into chronic skin infection. Inflammation and blindness will be the consequences through this infection. This disease causes through onchocerca volvulus parasite that is transmitted through a female black fly bite. This disease is also called as river blindness too. This infection will appear after one year to the black fly bite. There will be localized or general itching over the skin and this will result into scratching from the victim until skin breaks. This skin breakage will turn into small lumps over the skin. There will be fever, tiredness and headache too along with mentioned symptoms. Eye inflammation through this infection can lead to blindness. Nodules developed through this disease should be removed through surgery. It is a good choice to use ivermectin, which is capable enough to kill the parasite while symptoms started to appear over the victim.

**O'nyong-Nyong:** This is almost like dengue fever kind of infection found mostly in Asia and Africa. This disease transmitted to humans through anopheles mosquito bite and name suggests joints weakening in the dialect of Uganda. The symptoms associated with this disease are fever, severe pains to joints, swelling in lymph nodes and headache. There is no specific treatment for this disease, but antibiotics can be used for symptoms basing on their severity.

**Opportunistic Infection:** This infection is generally caused through harmless organisms and these organisms cannot infect healthy individuals. This infection will result into the people that are with weak resistance through diabetes or AIDS or cancer. Here, it is quite imperative to mention that long-term antibiotics usage can damage the immune system to result into a scope for the harmless organisms to turn into harmful too.

**Ornithosis:** This is also widely known as psittacosis or as parrot fever too. This disease generally transmitted to humans through infected exotic birds. This parrot fever causes through chlamydia psittaci bacteria found in most of the exotic birds. This fever resembles like pneumonia and blood test and patient history will be considered for diagnosis. Tetracycline is the right option to treat this parrot fever effectively. Patient is suggested to take acetaminophen, when fever is severed. If there is bad cough persistent, then suggested using codeine too.

**Osteomyelitis:** This is a bone and sometimes bone marrow infection and affects normally children long bones and vertebrae of adults. The chronic for of this disease will stay for years with constant flare-ups, when not treated properly. This disease is caused through staphylococci bacteria and this bacteria introduction will happen while surgery or trauma or through nearby infection or via bloodstream. There will be severe bone pain through this disease along with muscle spasm, tenderness, fever and headaches. Early stage of the disease will result into severe pain for the victim. It is essential to be on antibiotics for months along with bed rest for the victim. There is a chance for surgery too to stabilize infected bone through removal of affected bone and tissue.

**Otitis Externa:** This disease is also called as swimmer's ear too. This is an outer ear infection with inflammation. This is a generalized infection for ear through fungi or virus or bacteria or through trauma. There is a chance for the external era damage and ear canal damage through this disease. Rare cases will turn into malignant otitis externa too. Treatment for this disease is cleaning and keeping dry the affected area with antibiotics. You can add up some anti-inflammatory and anti-fungal drugs to the antibiotics for the quick and effective recovery. It is highly essential to keep the ear dry until recovered completely well. Badly swollen ear canal should be treated with nonprescription pain killers as the pain would be too severe.

**Otomycosis:** This is a fungal era infection also called as mycotic otitis externa too. This is a secondary bacterial infection causes through mycotic infection of ouet era canal along with A.Niger candida albicans or aspergillus fumigatus. This is a chronic and recurring infection. Treatment would be ideal with 5% aluminum acetate solution for swelling control along with Burrow's solution. Antifungal drops will add up well to this treatment too.

### Infectious Diseases Start with "P":

**Pandemic:** This is another widespread epidemic seen occurring all over the world.

**Papillomavirus, Human (HPV):** A group of virus with more than 70 varieties to cause into warts, genital warts, plantary warts and some more. This HPV virus got no cure.

**Paragonimiasis:** This is a disease causes through lung fluke, which is a pure parasitic flatworm. These parasitic worms will infect human that eats raw crab or the crayfish. This infection happens to humans, when handled or ate pickled crabs or raw crabs or crayfish. Mild infection will show no symptoms over the victims. The common symptoms associated with this disease are lung infestation with low fever along with dry cough. Slowly cough will turn into bloody cough. Victim will be weak, breath shortage, weight loss and fatigue once after cough turned into bloody. Many drugs are available to treat this disease and surgery is essential to remove formed cysts.

**Parainfluenza:** This is a respiratory virus to cause into respiratory infections for infants and children.

**Parasites:** Parasites are living things that are used to dwell within another living organism successfully. These parasites will live part or entire life within host through surviving with host contributes. Parasites nutritional requirements will be met through host tissues or blood or from host diet successfully. Some parasites are dangerous through carrying disease and interferes bodily functions and irritates tissues. Some will release toxins into the host body tissues. There are few human parasites like bacteria, fungus, protozoa, worms and viruses.

**Parasiticide:** This is an agent used to destroy parasites.

**Paratyphoid Fever:** This is a bacterial infection causes through salmonella bacteria.

**Paronychia:** This is an infection to skin at nail base area and it is caused through yeast called as candida albicans. Antibiotics and antifungal agents can treat this infection perfectly well.

**Parvovirus B 19:** This is a virus cause erythema infectiosum, which is a common childhood illness. This is also called as Fifth Disease and virus will present in mouth and nose secretions and blood.

**Pasteurella:** This bacilli genus to cause disease in animals and humans. This pasteurella infection transmits through animal bites to humans.

**Pasteurella Multocida:** This is a gram-negative species bacteria that can infect animals and this infection can be transmitted successfully to humans too via scratch or bite. This infection will result into wound or skin infection or blood poisoning. This bacterium generally resides within cat and dog mouth.

**Pasteurella Tularensis:** This is a verity of bacillus to cause into Tularemia.

**Pasteurellosis:** This bacterial disease generally transmitted to humans through dogs and cats. This disease causes through infected dog or cat bite or scratch. Dog bite very rarely to cause into infection as cat bite got more chances to result into infection in humans. It takes two days to show symptoms after the bite or scratch. Symptoms will be pain, redness, heat, and swelling. The glands near to wound will swell along with fever and chills. Lab test is right diagnosis procedure for this disease. This infection will be easily curable through Augmentin and people allergic to Pencillin can consider tetracycline.

**Pasteurization:** This is a process of applying heat up to a certain level to cheese or milk to kill the bacteria. Generally, milk pasteurization will need 145 to 150 degrees F.

**Pea Pickers' Disease:** This is a disease caused through lice as the lice feed over human blood in common. Lice are quick to transmit from one person to other. Most head lice infestation seen to happen in schools. The symptoms will start to appear within three weeks after infestation and turns into severe itching. The commonest infestation symptom is seen as scratching or itching over the area where lice feeding from human. Nowadays, many varieties of medicated shampoos, creams and rinses available to clear this problem successfully.

**Pelvic Inflammatory Disease:** This is an infection to the female reproductive organ like ovaries, fallopian tubes and uterus. There is no particular reason for this problem, but happens due to the untreated STD. like gonorrhea and chlamydia. Generally, bacteria will travel from the cervix to fallopian tubes, ovaries and uterus. Early stage of the disease will fail to show any symptoms, but progressive stage will show burning sensation while urinating, pelvic pain, severe cramps, heavy discharge during menstruation, and unusual discharge from vagina, low backache, fever, vomiting and nausea. Lab test through cervix sample culture can be a good diagnosis procedure to identify this disease. Intravenous antibiotic ointment along with hospitalization is required as a treatment for this disease. Mild conditions can be treated successfully a home with the help of antibiotics.

**Pencillin:** Pencillin was the first and foremost antibiotic developed for the humans. This was made from a mold and discovered by Alexander Fleming. This discovery resulted into a great help and support to develop many more antibiotics for humans. Pencillin is definitely a great gift to combat against the bacterial infections.

**Pets and Infectious Diseases:** Pets are definitely great companions for humans and help in many ways to relive stress in humans too. At the same time, there is few health risks too involved with pets for humans. Pets are some disease carriers and there is a long list of diseases to mention in this context and those are cat-scratch disease, Lyme disease, psittacosis, rabies, Rocky Mountain spotted fever, ringworm, roundworm, salmonellosis, strep throat, toxoplasmosis, and some more.

**Pfiesteria Picicida:** This one belongs to 450-million years old family. This one celled organism endures many life stages and few stages will release toxin that can easily penetrate into the human membranes. This toxin generally infested in waters and this will result into memory loss, disorientation, skin infections and some more dangers.

**Pharyngitis:** This is an cute infection to pharynx, which is a part between the throat tonsils and larynx. Viral infection is the major reason for this infection. This also can happen through mycoplasma or chlamydia bacteria too. Symptoms of this disease are almost similar to influenza or cold or diphtheria or scarlet fever. There will be sore throat with pain while swallowing and fever along with earache can be seen besides swelling to neck lymph nodes. Extensive swelling sometime can result into fluid buildup within larynx, which is too much dangerous for life. It is a good treatment for this disease to gargle warm salt water and bacterial infection will deserve usage of antibiotics for the effective treatment.

**Pinta:** This is a skin infection disease happens through treponema carateum organisms. This organism is a close relative to treponema palladium bacteria, which causes syphilis. This organism enters into the humans through breaking the skin. These diseases can transmit through prolonged or close contact with the infected person. This infection generally starts with a big spot that is surrounded with tiny spots over face or buttocks or neck or hands or feet. One year later, these spots will turn into red patches and eventually will transform into blue, brown and later to white. Swelling to lymph nodes may also take place with few victims. Pencillin G is the right treatment for this disease and tetracycline can also be a wise a choice too. Here, it is quite imperative to mention that the victims may sometimes disfigure due to this infection permanently.

**Pinworm Infestation:** This is another commonest parasitic infection for humans. This infection through pinworm is known as enterobiasis and generally this pinworm will reside within intestine of the humans. This pinworm will result into tickling for the infected person and this tickling sometimes can be seen as severe itching too. This infection generally occurs at anal area and itching sensation will be more during night time. This pinworm presence can be identified through microscope only. There are few ointments available to treat this infection and carbolated petroleum jelly can also be a good treatment too. It is suggested having sitz bath along with cleaning anal area with witch hazel.

**Plague:** Plague is serious infection disease and this is generally transmitted through rat fleas' bite. There are three disorders through this disease as bubonic, pneumonic and septicemic.

Each or together will attack the victim as a disease. Fleas are generally found over rodents and these fleas are got more chances to transmit this disease to humans. There are more than 100 varieties of flea species are found with plague virus. Symptoms will appear within five days after the infection. There will be sudden fever and some more symptoms basing on the type of disorder. Early stage of plague will be easy and successful for treatment. Here, untreated pneumonic plague is quite fatal and survival chances are almost slime. Treatment options are administering streptomycin, are you can try gentamicin, trimethoprim or sulfamethaxazole or chloramphenicol or tetracycline too.

**Plantar Warts:** These are hard, painful and rough-surface warts happen over sole of foot. This type of infection got chances to transmit to others through shower floors, when infected people walked over it. These warts are seen as soft with central core that is with firm ring like a callous. These warts generally disappear on own and few may stay for years and few will recur. There is no specific treatment for these warts.

**Plasmodium:** This is a genus belongs to protozoa and its four species known to be the reason for transmitting Malaria in humans via infected anopheles mosquito bite. This infection is also known as P. shigelloides too. This infection generally causes through tainted water and very often the organism found in swimming pools unsanitary water or in drinking water or while food items rinsed in these types waters. This P.shigelloides gastroenteritis is completely self-limiting disease. The symptoms will be fever, abdominal pain, chills, watery diarrhea, nausea and vomiting. These symptoms will appear after eating or drinking water that is with mentioned organisms. Bacteriological analysis is needed to diagnosis this disease in victims.

**Pneumococcal Vaccine:** This is a vaccine to prevent the dangerous pneumococcal pneumonia. It is a safe vaccine with cost effective pricing.

**Pneumococcus:** This pneumococcal disease will attack elderly or people with serious medical conditions like kidney problems, heart problems, lung problems and some more. This pneumococcus is also called as streptococcus too. This is transmitted through airborne from person to person. Symptoms will start to appear within three days after the infection. Symptoms will be fever, headache, chills, cough, disorientation, chest pain, stiff neck and shortage of breath. Specific lab test is essential to diagnosis of the disease through culture of sputum, spinal fluid or blood. Pencillin or cephalosporin should be administered promptly to the victims as a treatment. Some of the pneumococcus strains are resistant with Pencillin and require strong medication for complete eradication.

**Pneumonia:** It is an infection to the lungs and this is one of the dangerous infectious diseases that can lead to death to the victim. This is termed as influenza common complication. This Pneumonia can cause in various forms as parasitic, bacterial, viral, fungal and mycoplasmic. This pneumonia is generally caused through microorganism inhaling and chances are there for the germ to reach lung via bloodstream too. Symptoms are shaking chills, cough with colored discharge, fever, chest pain, and inflammation in lungs. Antibiotics like Pencillin can be a right treatment for the bacterial pneumonia. Antibiotics will be more effective, when considered during early stage.

**Pneumonia, Bacterial:** Pneumonia or lung infection or lung inflammation causes through S.pneumoniae bacteria or staphycoccus aureus or klebsiella pneumoniae or pseudomonas aeruginosa or haemophillus influenza or legionella pneumophilla or mycoplasma pneumoniaea bacteria. This infection will start with sudden severe chills and racing fever along with chest pain, troubled breathing and cough. Blood test, x-ray and culture can diagnosis this disease very well for the victim. Antibiotics are right solution for treating this infection and Pencillin G will work well too. There are few more drugs that are proven to be effective with disease are erythromycin, the cephalosporin, clindamycin, trimethoprim-sulfamethoxazole and other Pencillins.

**Pneumonia, Chlamydial:** This is a novice pneumonia caused through new discovered member of chlamydia. This infection was earlier named as Taiwan Acute Respiratory agent pneumonia. This chlamydia pneumonia causes through tiny organism known as chlamydia pneumonia. This infection can transmit to others by direct contact with infected individual or through breathing bacteria while infected person coughing. Symptoms are similar to other types of pneumonia like sore throat, fatigue, fever, cough and weakness. Tetracycline or erythromycin can be suitable antibiotics to treat this infection effectively. These medicines wil clear the infection within 21 days successfully.

**Pneumonia, Pneumococcal:** This pneumococcal pneumonia causes through streptococcus pneumoniae bacteria and this infection spreads through air or through exposing directly with respiratory drops of a person that was already infected. Symptoms will start within three days after the infection with fever, headache, chills, chest pain, cough, breathing problems, and stiff neck. This disease is generally diagnosed through symptoms and sputum culture, spinal fluid and blood culture. Antibiotics can clear this disease effectively.

**Pneumonia, Pneumocystis Carini:** This PCP is also called as AIDS pneumonia too. This disease is prone to the people that are with weak immune system. This disease causes through pneumocystis carini species and spreads successfully through air, personal contact, and through infected person cough and breathing. The symptoms are breathing trouble, fever, dry cough, nail beds and lips will turn into blue, and these symptoms will be there up to few months. Sputum or lung biopsy is required for the diagnosis of this disease. This is a fatal infection and can be treated successfully with high doses of antibiotics like cotrimoxazole.

**Poliomyelitis:** This is a contagious virus disease and this disease severe form will result into paralysis for the victims. This disease causes through three different types of viruses that are clearly present in intestinal tract, nose and throat. Here, people are perfect carriers of this disease to infect others. It can spread easily hand to hand and other contacts. Symptoms will be fever, nausea, sore throat, stomach ache and head ache. Specific treatment is not yet available and recovery mainly varies significantly from one to other basing on so many other factors.

**Pork and Infectious Diseases:** Pork that is undercooked can cause many different varieties of infectious diseases to humans. Some of those are listeriosis, yersiniosis, trichinosis and pork tapeworm or taeniasis.

**Poultry and Infectious Diseases:** Poultry that is undercooked can result into many types of infectious diseases. Some of these for example are yersiniosis and salmonellosis. This poultry should be suggested cooking up to 180 degrees F or up to the juices will be cleared successfully.

**Pregnancy and Infectious Diseases:** There are some of the infectious diseases that can be contracted through pregnant woman and some of these diseases will be harmful for the unborn child too. Some of those diseases are chicken pox, chlamydia, cytomegalovirus, fifth disease, genital herpes, genital warts, German measles, gonorrhea, Group B Strep, Hepatitis B, AIDS, Japanese encephalitis, listeriosis, Lyme disease, malaria, shingles, syphilis, toxoplasmosis, and trichomoniasis.

**Prion:** This is an unusual and different type of infection agent. It looks like neither bacteria nor virus. It has no genetic material. This prion is comprised of protein causes disease like Creutzfeldt-Jakob disease to human brain, and the same disorder can be seen in cows, sheep and other animals too. This infection agent been implicated in mad cow disease too. There is still no specific treatment available to treat this infection.

**Prostatitis:** This disease can be seen in the chronic and acute forms and results into inflammation to prostate glands. It can happen through bacteria, mycoplasma infection or through fungal. This prostatitis happens through an infection that has initiated from urethra. It may be or may not be a STD too. Symptoms will be urination with burning sensation along with frequent urination urge. There is a chance for blood discharge through penis due to this infection.

Acute condition will cause fever, low back ache, abdominal pain and cough. Antibiotics can heal this infection successfully and it is suggested having sitz bath, more fluids and bed rest.

**Protegrin:** It is a variety of peptide that is offering wide-spectrum for microbial treatments derived for many types of infectious diseases. This can be of great help to treat some of the diseases that are quite resistant with antibiotics.

**Protozoa:** This protozoon is a simple and one cell animal life. This protozoa means is a "first animals' too. This single animal successfully carries out all required life functions successfully. This animal like organism gets required nutrient from surrounding environment successfully.

**Pseudomembranous Enterocolitis:** This is a diarrheal disease and known as hospital-acquired infection too. This disease is generally associated with antibiotic therapy. It will develop due to the toxin production and overgrowth through C. difficile within the body colon. Symptoms are different types of diarrhea along with dehydration, cramps, nausea, and abdominal distention. Diagnosis of this disease will be confirmed through finding C.difficile toxin within the patient stool sample. Therapy should be initiated at the early stage with electrolyte replacement and fluids and discontinue antibiotics that are resulted into this disease.

**Pseudomonas Aeruginosa:** This is another gram-negative bacteria generally isolated from blood, wounds, sputum, infections and burns related to urinary tract. These bacteria are quite resistant with antibiotics and disinfectants.

**Psychiatric Disease and Infections:** Human central nervous system is always susceptible to various infections. There are few varieties of mental disorders that are very well connected with certain infectious agents. Some of those are AIDS dementia, manic depression, schizophrenia, and obsessive compulsive disorder.

**Pyelonephritis:** this is a bacterial infection to kidneys to cause inflammation. The acute pyelonephritis will happen through bladder infection that will successfully spread up to kidney. The chronic version will happen during childhood due to urine flow back into ureters. This kind of urine flow can result into recurring kidney infection for the victim. Symptoms are high fever, back pain and chills. There is a possibility for this infection to lead into septicemia too and antibiotics can be a good treatment for this disease and administered intravenously.

**Infectious Diseases Start with "Q"**

**Q fever:** This is a respiratory illness for animals and this called as Australian Q fever too. This animal fever can be easily transmitted to humans from domestic and pet animals. This disease generally happens through coxiella burnetii bacteria. This disease spread through infected domestic and pet animals. This disease also happens through contaminated milk or through infected tick bite too. Symptoms will be high fever, chills, fatigue, muscle pain, headache, weakness, and sweating and chest pain. Blood test can reveal the antibodies successfully and this right diagnosis procedure to identify this disease. There are few antibiotics like tetracycline can result well against this disease. Chronic disease will deserve sage of antibiotics for long-term.

## Infectious Diseases Start with "R"

**Rabies:** Rabies is an acute viral disease to the human central nervous system. This disease is generally transmitted through the bite of an infected warm-blood animal. Untreated rabies can be quite deadly to humans. It is highly essential to have vaccine immediately after the animal bite. Rabies happens through viral encephalitis and transmitted to humans through the infected animal saliva. This infection can affect badly spine and brain of the victim. Symptoms are having chance to appear between 10 and 50 days after the animal bite. Symptoms will appear mild in human and turns into wild and drastic down the line. Victim will more restless, anxious, excitable, and irritable. There will be insomnia and depression too. There will be hallucination and victim will salivate along with pain and muscle spasm in throat. Currently, there are proving tests for rabies in lab and it should be identified through the down the line symptoms. Treatment is to wash the wound immediately, when a rabid animal bites human. Let the wound bleed in a way it can washout on own. There is rabies vaccine to treat the problem, but this should be administered only after virus exposure.

**Rash in Infectious Diseases:** Rashes will happen through many reasons like drug reaction, allergy, insect bites, and some more. Here, some of the infectious diseases also will cause rashes. For example, rash due to fever is an infectious disease. Similarly, there are wide varieties of infectious rashes can appear like through measles, chicken pox, German measles, and some more.

**Rat-Bite Fever:** This is a fever causes through rat bite. This disease generally transmitted to humans by rats and there is a chance to transmit the same through squirrels, wild mice and weasels too. There are two types of bacteria being culprit to cause into this disease and those are streptobacillus moniliformis and spirillum minus. Symptoms will be sudden fever, headache, chills and muscle ache. There will be joint pains too, when the disease happens through streptobacillus moniliformis. Blood culture can reveal this disease successfully in the lab. Pencillin is always a wise treatment for this disease and pain killers can be added to it to get relief from fever and other symptoms.

**Rats and Infectious Diseases:** Rodents always live close and around to humans. These rodents are real health threat for humans in many ways. Rats always a great reason for spreading many dangerous diseases to humans. Plague and typhus are main diseases to be mentioned in this context as these will transmit to humans by rodents. Rat bite fever doesn't require special mentioning as name itself is indicating everything.

**Red Tide:** Red tide happens through toxic plankton and shellfish requires special mentioning as these fish live through plankton and turns into contaminated to result into dangerous for humans. Red tides are mainly seen in coastal waters.

**Relapsing Fever:** This relapsing fever causes through spirochete borrelia and transmitted successfully to humans through lice and ticks. There will be sudden fever due to this disease along with chills, headache, muscle pain and vomiting. There is a chance for rash over legs and arms too. Later stage can lead into jaundice too. This disease diagnosis is carried out through finding spirochete in the blood smear. Treatment for this disease can be effective with Pencillin, chloramphenicol and tetracycline.

**Reovirus:** Reovirus is one that is with three types virus with double stranded RNA. These viruses generally cause upper respiratory tract infections and sometimes infantile gastroenteritis.

**Reportable Disease:** Contagious diseases are always supposed to be reported to family physician or to public health authorities. This will result into immediate report to the Center for Disease Control and Prevention. Public health officers can take necessary measures in a way diseases will be controlled and prevented successfully from transmitting to others.

**Respiratory Syncytial Virus (RSV) Infection:** This is a respiratory illness caused through myxovirus. This RSV generally transmits through contact from the infected person nose and throat droplets. Also, it can transmit through sneeze and cough of the infected person too. Symptoms will be severe pneumonia along with cough, wheezing, fatigue and running nose. This RSV generally diagnosed through symptoms and severe illness needs lab testing. There is no specific treatment for this disease, but bed rest and clear fluids can help to recover well. Children with disease can be treated with antiviral drug like ribavirin during early stage.

**Respiratory Tract Infections:** Infections happened to upper or lower respiratory tract will result into so many health problems. Upper respiratory tract infection can cause cold, pharyngitis, laryngitis, rhinitis, tonsillitis and sinusitis. Lower respiratory tract infection can cause bronchitis, pneumonia, bronchiolitis, lung abscess, tuberculosis, emphysema and some more.

**Retrovirus:** This is an RNA virus like HIV, which cause into AIDS.

**Rheumatic Fever:** This is an inflammatory disease happens through untreated beta-hemolytic streptococcal infection that belongs to the upper respiratory tract. There is a chance for this rheumatic fever due to the untreated scarlet fever and strep throat. Symptoms will be fever, nose bleeding, joint pains, stomach ache, and nausea. There will be chest pain too with some cases along with heart problems. Diagnosis of rheumatic fever is hard as it resembles like many other illnesses. It is diagnosed through symptoms as joint pain, chorea, carditis, rash and fever. Pencillin is so far suggested medication to treat rheumatic fever and add this with steroids basing on the severity of disease.

**Rhinitis, Viral:** This is an infection to the mucous membrane nose lining happens through virus. This can lead into sinusitis as this infection cause nasal obstruction sneezing, facial pain and nasal discharge.

**Rhinoscleroma:** This is a bacterial infection happens through klebsiella rhinoscleromatis. Symptoms will be severe nasal secretion along with crusting. There is a chance for upper lip and nose enlargement too through this infection. This infection slowly reaches to upper respiratory down the line to result into breathing problems. This is a difficult disease to treat effectively and requires systemic antibiotics like tobramycin and gentamicin. There is a need for oral administration of ciprofloxacin is also needed for the effective treatment.

**Rhinovirus:** Rhino virus is with more than 200 distinct varieties in it and causes around 40% of respiratory illnesses. Symptoms of this infection will be scratchy dry throat, headache, malaise, and nasal congestion. There will be fever along with nasal discharge for two days and children will suffer with cough. Treatment is available to offer relief from symptoms only and try using painkillers, nasal decongestant and antihistamines. There is a chance to reduce the illness to short duration through using vitamin c and zinc.

**Rickettsia Akari:** This is parasite lives over insects and animals like lice, fleas and mites. This will carry typhus.

**Rickettsial Infections:** This disease will transmit through feces or bites of insects that are carrying parasitic organisms known as rickettsia. The diseases caused through this infection are Rocky Mountain spotted fever, q fever and some varieties of typhus. This rickettsia is a tiny bacteria and capable enough to invade cells of any other live-form through multiplying quickly.

**Rickettsial Pox:** This is an urban diseases cause through the bite of house mouse or a mite. The bacteria reason for this disease is rickettsia akari.

**Rickettsia Prowazekki:** this is a parasite lives over insects and some animals like mites, lice, fleas and ticks.

**Rickettsia Rickettsii:** This is an intercellular parasite organism and looks almost like a tiny bacteria. These parasites will reproduce through invading into the cells of any other live-form. These parasites will live over insects and few animals and these insects and animals will infect domestic animals, pets and humans.

**Rickettsia Tsutsugamushi:** This is a parasite lives over insects and tiny animals such as lice and some more.

**Rift Valley Fever:** this is a virus transmitted disease and virus is known as aedes. It will transmit through mosquitoes. Symptoms are similar dengue fever and starts with high fever, headache, and visual problems. There will be fatal bleeding too with rare cases. Treatment is purely symptomatic.

**Ringworm (tinea):** This is a skin infection happens through fungus and affects skin, scalp, fingers, feet and toenails. This ringworm spreads through skin to skin contact via infected people, pets and indirect contact via shower stalls, barber clips, and floors. Symptoms will begin with tiny pimple, which will turn into bigger with scaly patches over scalp. Ringworm to scalp is known as tinea captis and seen with temporary bald patches and dandruff scales. Microscopic inspection can reveal the presence of ringworm for the infected individual. Treatment is ideal with antifungal medication like griseofulvin. Antifungal ointment application over the affected area can stop spreading to further extent too.

**Risus Sardonicus:** this is an unusual form of grinning expression causes due to prolonged contraction of facial muscles. Sometimes this kind of problem can be seen as a symptom with tetanus too.

**Rocky Mountain spotted fever:** This is another infectious disease identified through spotted rash. This RMSF will spread through the bite of infected dog tick or through lone-star tick or through wood tick. There is a chance for this infection through contamination of skin via feces or tick blood too. Symptoms will be fever for three weeks along with losing appetite, headache, and some more. There will be pink spots within six days after the infection over ankle and wrist and spreads all over the body down the line. This will subside on own within two weeks. Diagnosis is difficult with this infection as symptoms will resemble with many other simalr diseases. Blood and tissue test at lab can be a good help in this context. Antibiotics will be the right treatment for this infection and doxycycline or tetracycline will be right choice. You can try chloramphenicol too.

**Roseola (Exanthem subitum):** This is an infectious disease commonly happens during childhood. Symptoms will be irritability, fever, rash and some more. Symptoms will come and go occasionally for few days. There is no specific lab test available to confirm roseola. There is no complication associated with this disease and acetaminophen can be used to reduce the fever.

**Rotavirus:** This virus every year striking more than 130 million people all over the world. Around 870,000 children are dying through this dangerous virus every year worldwide. Rotavirus generally invades cell that belongs to the small bowel to absorb its liquids. This will result into diarrhea for the victim. Rotavirus not alone infects humans and it can attack animals too. Symptoms will be vomiting, low fever, and watery diarrhea up to 8 days. This is infectious in children until diarrhea stops or controlled. Symptoms are the only possibility to diagnosis this infection. Treatment for rotavirus is not available and it is strictly instructed not to use any nonprescription diarrhea drugs to infected children and infants. There is a great necessity for IV-fluid replacement for children with severe dehydration.

**Roundworms:** These are also known as nematodes and these are cylindrical worms with more than 12 types in it. These are parasites on humans. Symptoms will be zero with adult worms that are resided within the human intestines. There will be few symptoms, when worm larvae reach certain parts of the body. This worm infestation or worm burden can be relieved through anthelmintic drugs.

## Infectious Diseases Start with "S"

**Salmonella Bacteria:** This is a type of bacteria, which in general causes food poisoning called as salmonellosis. This will include S. choleraesuis, salmonella entertidis, S. aertrycke and S. cubana. These bacteria type is famous multiplying fast at common room temperature and very commonly seen in raw meat, fish, eggs, poultry, raw milk and other foods made of these items. Also, these bacteria present in pet turtles too. The S.Typhe bacterium that belongs to Salmonella family is most dangerous and causes into typhoid fever for humans.

**Salmonellosis:** This is a major type of food poisoning through bacteria. This salmonellosis is not dangerous, but mostly one percent of cases can turn into fatal. This food poisoning can happen through salmonella bacteria and surprising fact is that the low dose of these bacteria that is hard to identify can result into reasonable food poisoning successfully. Symptoms will start to appear within 2 days. This can happen through consuming tainted food, tainted marijuana, touching infected turtles, and some more. Symptoms will vary basing on the amount of bacteria attacked through the contaminated items. There will be headache, vomiting, nausea, stomach cramps, fever and diarrhea. Some types of food poisoning currently do not have specific treatment. There will be dehydration through this food poisoning and this should be combated through taking plenty of fluids and bland diet. There are few antibiotics to try against this problem such as ampicillin or chloramphenicol or tetracycline. Antibiotics administration is suggested only, when bacteria found in blood.

**Scabies:** This is a common skin infestation and highly infectious too. This infection causes through mite sarcoptes scabiel, which enters into the skin and lays eggs. These scabies mites generally pass through personal contact, passes through bed sheets or underwear used by infected people, and some more ways. Symptoms will be severe itching and this will be more intense during nights. There will be swelling with gray patches over genitals, wrist breast, nipples, thighs, lower buttocks and in arm pits. There will be lumps down the line over trunk and limbs. Treatment will be insecticide lotion like lindane, crotamiton or permethrin. This lotion can kill mites successfully and apply it all over the skin. There will be itching continuation for 2 weeks after usage of the lotion, but suggested continuing the lotion usage for the entire family.

**Scarlet Fever:** This is a childhood bacterial infectious disease. There will fever, skin rash and sore throat to the victim through this disease. Scarlet fever mainly spreads through bacteria. This can transmit through droplets of the infected person cough or sneeze or breathe. This can also transmit from the infected person through sharing food and drink too. Incubation period will be 4 days with disease and first illness will start to appear over the victim. There will be severe fever along with sore throat. Face will be flushed along with red spots and white coating over the tongue. Treatment for this disease will be antibiotics course for ten days with erythromycin or

Pencillin. Children with this disease will be contagious up to 2 days after initiating the treatment too and later will be totally free from being contagious.

**Schistosomiasis:** This is an infection causes through flukes that multiply and live within freshwater snails. Initially, this parasite will infect snails and release huge volume of larvae into the water. These larvae will reach into humans through gaining entry via unbroken skin. These larvae will grow into adults within the host and these adults eggs will result into inflammatory reactions for the humans. The parasites will slowly start to reach intestine and liver via blood. Symptoms will appear within 3 weeks after the infection. Skin will experience dermatitis, lesions and hives. The latest drug praziquantel is a perfect treatment for this infection. Single dose of this drug can kill all the flukes successfully and prevents damage. Other alternative drugs are metriphonate and oxamniquine.

**Scrofula:** This scrofula is a former term to tuberculosis of lymphatic glands and bones. This is also called as king's evil too.

**Septicemia (Bacterial sepsis):** This is a medical name for the blood poisoning and quite fatal one too. This septicemia causes through certain types bacteria, when entered into the bloodstream. These bacteria will release toxin called endotoxins, which is a dangerous poisonous substance. This poison can stay after the bacteria disintegration too and results into drop with blood pressure along with rapid breathing and heartbeat. Symptoms will be fever, diarrhea, chills, headache, rapid breathing, and nausea. Septicemia can be diagnosed through blood culture in lab. Antibiotics are the perfect option to treat this problem along with IV fluids. It is highly imperative to identify the site of infection and requires surgical removal too.

**Septic Shock:** This is a type of shock happens through drop in blood pressure and through tissue damage. This kind of situation generally happens through septicemia blood poisoning and toxemia. This shock in general follows with severe infection to humans. This problem is mainly due to the toxins released into the bloodstream of the infected individual. This toxin can damage sell and cause into blood pressure drop to a significant extent. Symptoms will be dependent over the tissue damage status. General symptoms will be as similar as septicemia along with cold hands and feet, weak pulse, blood pressure drop and blue coloration. Septic shock deserves immediate treatment through fluid replacement and with antibiotics. Surgery is also essential to remove the infected portion within the body.

**Sexually Transmitted Diseases (STD):** Any type of contagious disease that is having scope to transmit through sexual intercourse or through general contact is termed as STD. This STD is also known as venereal disease too. This STD quite normally seen with people those are with multiple sex partners. Some types of STD have scope to transmit through blood and chances to acquire through drug addicts that commonly shares needles.

**Shellfish Poisoning:** Shellfish eating can lead into so many types of diseases similar to bacterial or virus or toxin infectious diseases. Shellfish got more scope for viral and bacterial contamination. This is due to their living atmosphere that is close to shore, which is more prone to pollution. Originally shellfish is not poisonous, but contaminated due to so many factors around to its living area.

**Shellfish Poisoning, Amnesic:** Amnesic shellfish poisoning will happen through unusual neurotoxin that is domoic acid or amino acid, which generally contaminates a shellfish successfully. This toxin generally created within shellfish due to their habit to eat phytoplankton. Symptoms of this amnesic shellfish poisoning will dangerous neurological effects start to appear within a day after eating this fish. Symptoms will be diarrhea, abdominal pain, vomiting, memory loss, confusion, seizure, disorientation and coma. There is no suitable lab test to diagnosis this problem and it should be identified through symptoms alone. There is no suitable antidote for this poisoning and treatment should be considered to ease the symptoms.

**Shellfish Poisoning, Diarrhea:** This shellfish poisoning diarrhea will cause through eating contaminated shellfish and its toxin-producing plankton. This poisoning can also happen through eating oysters, mussels and scallops too. Symptoms will start to appear within 3 hours after eating contaminated fish. There will be gastrointestinal problems along with muscle weakness, headache, chills, and fever. Symptoms and diet history are the options to diagnosis this problem. There is no suitable antidote for this poisoning and recovery will happen on own.

**Shellfish Poisoning, Neurotoxic:** This neurotoxic shellfish poisoning happens through group of toxins known as brevetoxins. There will be gastrointestinal problems and neurological problems through this poisoning. The symptoms will start to appear within few minutes after eating the contaminated shellfish. There will be tingling along with numbness to tongue, lip and throat, muscle pains, dizziness, sensation reversal, vomiting and diarrhea. This sould be diagnosed through symptoms alone. There is no specific treatment for this poisoning and drugs are available to ease the symptoms.

**Shellfish Poisoning, paralytic (PSP):** There are twenty varieties of toxins those can lead into PSP and these are all derivatives of saxitoxin. This saxitoxin is capable enough to interfere with brain functions, senses and movements. Symptoms will appear within few minutes. There will be numbness to tongue along with tingling. Down the line, this numbness will spread to fingertips, and toes along with nausea, and headache. There will be additional symptoms like diarrhea and vomiting too. Lab tests cannot determine the PSO and it should be diagnosed through symptoms and diet history. There is no antidote for PSP and suggested administering prostigmine along with artificial oxygen and respiration. It is a good option to induce vomiting too, which can help to eliminate remaining toxin contained shellfish from the body.

**Shigellosis:** This is a bacteria diarrhea through shigella bacteria. This shigella bacterium is comprised of four species in it. Symptoms will take 8 hours and in some cases 8 days to appear. There will be nausea, watery diarrhea, vomiting, stomach cramps, vision problems, weakness headache and swallowing issues. People with weak immune system will experience severe diarrhea. Stool culture is the right diagnosis procedure to locate this disease. Recovery generally happens on own, but fluids replacement will be ideal to avoid dehydration. Antibiotics usage can help well to shorten the diarrhea and disease to a significant extent.

**Shingles:** This is a red blistering painful viral infection to the nerves. Chickenpox virus will be dormant after treatment within sensory nerves along with spine. This dormant virus will be active once again, when immune system weakened and reaches into the skin through receptor ends. There will be an initial symptom with pain in the skin and rashes will appear after 5 days. These rashes will turn into yellow blisters down the line in few days. The nerves will experience damage through this virus attack and blisters heal will not be of any help as the damaged nerves keep on paining a lot for the victim. This pain will endure for months to years. Antiviral drugs are the best option for treating this problem. There are few best proven antiviral drugs like famcyclovir, acyclovir and valacyclovir. It is always a good option to seek medical attention immediately after witnessing the first sign of shingles.

**Sin Nombre Virus:** This is newest strain that belongs to Hantavirus.

**Sinusitis:** This is a type of inflammation to one or sometimes more of sinuses, which can turn into a complication for the respiratory as infection or as dental infection. This problem also can happen due to allergies or due to air travel or due to underwater swimming. This sinusitis causes through spreading infection from nose and its narrow passage that drains mucous. This will result into swelling to mucous membranes and blocks the openings from sinuses to nose. This blockage will turn into building up secretion of sinus and teams up with bacteria down the line. There is a chance for this infection to happen through abscess too. Symptoms will be pressure, headache, local tenderness, fever, and tension. Stuffy nose resulted through this problem can lose the ability to smell too. There is a chance to locate the disorder through x-Ray and culture may be grown from sinus swab to identify the resided bacteria. Steam inhalation, antibiotics, nasal decongestants, and painkillers can be the right treatment for this problem. Surgery also can be a wise choice to improve the drainage and ideal for chronic issues.

**Skin Infections:** Skin is always an outer barrier to human with the outer world. I will defend the interior body from the possible attackers like bacteria, insect venom, viruses, and fungi. These skin infections generally range from superficial problems like impetigo to many types of widespread fatal infections.

**Sleeping Sickness:** This is also known as African trypanosomiasis, which is another serious infectious disease for tropical Africa. This disease causes through parasites that are transmitted via bite of the infected tsetse flies. This disease is mainly widespread among animals and rare in humans. Painful nodule will develop at the place, where fly bitten to the victim and this will progress slowly along with fever and enlargement to lymph glands. Parasites slowly will invade blood vessels of the victim to damage central nervous system. The symptoms will be drowsiness, sleepiness and lethargy. Untreated patients with this disease will die too. Blood, cerebrospinal fluid or lymph fluid should be tested through microscope for the parasites presence as a part of diagnosis. The drug named as suramin can treat this disease effectively.

**Smallpox:** This is another serious infectious viral disease. This smallpox is completely eradicated through international cooperative vaccine program. This disease happens only to humans and victims will be easy to recognize and will be infectious short-time.

**Sore Throat:** The throat with pain and scratchy feeling along with cold or through other types of infection is called sore throat and causes through organisms. It is not a serious issue and an indication to the bacterial infection.

**Spinal Tap:** This is also known as lumbar puncture and it is a procedure to remove cerebrospinal fluid with the help of hollow needle. This procedure will help to diagnosis the infectious diseases and spinal tap is real help for many infectious diseases identification and treatment.

**Spirochetes:** these spirochetes are slender bacterial organisms and considered protozoa too.

**Sporotrichosis:** This is a chronic fungal infection to skin and it follows very often trauma with painful ulcers and abscesses. This is caused through sporothrix schenckii bacteria. This disease very commonly appears with nursery workers those are commonly handle sphagnum moss or thorny plants or baled hay. There will be several forms of disorders through this infection like acute skin problems, painless bumps, and many more. This disease is confirmed in the lab through fungus culture from the swab of pus or biopsy fresh bump skin. Treatment for this problem is potassium iodide droplets for 6 weeks. There is a drug too available to treat this problem known as itraconazole. Flucytosine or amphotericin also can be sued.

**St. Anthony's fire:** This is also called as erysipelas and it is a fatal streptococcal infection to the skin with oozing swellings over face with headache and blistering. Severe cases will deserve hospitalization and antibiotics intravenous administration.

**Staphylococcal Infections:** There are several types of infections to cause through staphylococcal bacteria and most of these infections characterized through formation of abscesses over skin and other organs. Most of these infections treatment includes bed rest, antimicrobial drug, painkillers and surgical drainage.

**Staphylococcal Scalded Skin Syndrome:** This is a type of blistering skin rash commonly seen in newborns due to toxins released through staphylococcal bacteria. This disease is very much prone to infants that are with weak immunity or with kidney problems. Symptoms will be skin rash that resemble like a burn along with blistering and skin peeling to result into scalded look. There is a great necessity to administer antistaphylococcal antibiotics for the victim as a treatment. Skin should be kept under cover with dressing and antibiotic ointments like bacitracin.

**Sterilization:** This is a procedure to eliminate completely or destruct all types of microbial life. It is essential to keep hospitals, and hospital equipment completely sterilized with the help of steam or dry heat or through liquid chemicals.

**Strep Throat (Streptococcal Pharyngitis):** This is a throat infection causes through bacteria known as beat-hemolytic streptococcus. Here, people with group A strep and nasal passages can be healthy and with more scope to spread the disease to others that are actively ill.

Most of the cases will have no symptoms through this disease and some will experience within 3 days after infection. There will be high fever, swelling with throat, and some more. This is a viral infection and requires lab test to confirm as a part of diagnosis practice. Antibiotics are the proven wise treatment against the positive strep throat. Antibiotics should be continued for a week as chances are here for this disease to turn into rheumatic fever,

**Sterptobacillus Moniliformis:** This is a bacteria shaped as necklace and causes rat-bite fever in humans.

**Streptococcal Infections:** Streptococcal infections are caused through a group of bacteria and it is a most common bacteria group to cause various types of infections to humans. Some variety of strep bacteria will always exist in human throat harmlessly. Some type of strep bacteria can lead into sore throat, era infections, tonsillitis, pneumonia and strep throat.

**Streptococcus:** This is a gram-positive bacterium happens to be in pairs or in the form of short chain or chains. Many of these species can cause certain types of infectious diseases for humans.

**Streptococcus, Group A (GAS):** Most of the strep illness forms will develop due to the group-A strep bacteria. This invasive GAS disease may occurs, when bacteria succeeds past to the immune defenses. These germs got chances to spread through contact with throat and nose discharge or through coming in contact with infected lesions over the skin. The intensity of infection will be more, when it transmitted through infected would and while ill. Treatment of

GAS is possible with the help of proven antibiotics like pencillin. Erythromycin can be a choice for the people that are allergic to Pencillin.

**Streptococcus, Group B (GBS):** This is an illness happens to pregnant women, infants, and elderly through Group-B bacteria of streptococcus. This is a most commonly seen blood infection and meningitis for newborns. Most of humans will carry GBS bacteria in their bodies in the places like bowels, urinary tract, genitals, lungs or throat. 40% of pregnant women will have these bacteria in vagina or in rectum. Symptoms in infants would be seen within few hours after the birth. There is a chance for this disease in infant after few months to the birth too. Diagnosis of this disease can be identified through blood or spinal fluid culture in the lab. Treatment for this problem is antibiotics like ampicillin and Pencillin.

**Streptococcus Pneumoniae:** These are more than 70 types of pneumococci bacteria that can result into pneumonia in humans. These bacteria are resistant to Pencillin from moderate and high.

**Strongylodiasis:** This is an intestinal infestation through small roundworm parasites. This will cause itching and red patches over the skin from, where bacteria gained entry into the body. This disease happens through strongyloides stercoralis bacteria. There will be symptoms after infestation as redness, hives, itching, swelling and these will clear off in two days automatically. Thiabendazole is a promising drug to treat this disease efefctively.

**Sulfonamides (Sulfa Drug):** Synthetic drugs in large groups are used to treat many types of bacterial infections and these are derived from red dye or sulfanilamide. These drugs are quite effective to control the bacterial growth and will not kill bacteria. These drugs are used as combination with some other to treat some varieties of conditions like bronchitis, urinary tract infection, pneumonia, era infections, skin infections, and many more. There are few side effects involved with the usage of sulfonamides like jaundice, anemia, when consumed more than 10 days.

**Sweating Sickness, English:** This is a contagious disease that was more rampant during 15th century. The sweating through this disease resembles like scarlet fever and pneumonia. This sweating will strike almost for 24 hours with profuse sweating condition from head to toe along with back ache, pains in shoulder, head, legs, arms and intestinal problems. This disease is capable enough to kill the victim within two hours duration too.

**Swimmer's Itch:** This is also known as schistosomiasis or also called as cercarial dermatitis too. This will cause through the flatworms bite to result into inflammation to skin along with itching. These flatworms generally transmitted into the water through mammals or birds. Itchy feeling will start and lasts for one hour after coming in contact with the water that is contaminated with schistosomes worms. Flukes will successfully enter into the skin in this one hour duration. There will be swelling along with time red macule and this will transform into itchy papules in 15 hours. Other symptoms will vary basing on the sensitivity of the infected victim. There is no specific diagnosis procedure available to identify this disease due to various other issues. There is no specific treatment, but suggested using Calamine lotion or antithistamines oral medicine to control itching. Symptoms will stay up to 3 days and disappear on own.

**Syphilis:** This is STD happens through rash or skin sore. Syphilis generally causes through spirochete trepnema pallidum bacteria that enter through broke skin or through the mucous membranes during sex. Sore appeared during first stage of syphilis will take 4 weeks of time and this sore will have hard painless base and clears within a month. This sore happens over penis shaft for male and for female it will happen over labia. Pencillin is a proven wise treatment for syphilis, but treatment will be more effective, when considered at early stage.

**Infectious Diseases Start with "T"**

**Tapeworm:** This is a worm belongs to the Cestoda class and it is an intestinal worm. There are three different species of tapeworms and these tapeworms acquire humans when eaten up undercooked or raw contaminated fish or meat. There are different varieties of tapeworms to result into disease for humans as beef tapeworm, pork tapeworm, and fish tapeworm.

**T cell:** This is a type of white blood cell and also known as lymphocyte too. This cell is very much involves in the body cellular immune response. There will be helper T cells to activate other T cells. These T cells are the major target for HIV virus to result into AIDS.

**Tetanus:** Tetanus is fatal and acute infectious disease also known as "lockjaw" too. This disease generally happens to jaw muscles to result into lock. There is a vaccine for this disease and administered during childhood. It is essential to consider boosters too for the virus otherwise would be a risk. This disease caused through clostridium family bacteria and these bacteria can thrive successfully within the absence of oxygen. This will transmit through puncture wounds and through animal contact. Sometimes ear infection can lead to a rare form of tetanus too. This tetanus is capable enough to attack the central nervous system of the human through producing rigidity to muscles along with muscle spasm. Symptoms start to appear within three weeks after the infection and incubation period is estimated to be up to 50 days. Shorter incubation period cases are more prone to death. Symptoms will be headache, muscular stiffness, irritability, jaw and neck lock and some more. Treatment for this disease is powerful tranquilizers along with antispasmodic drugs. Generally, symptoms will be there with the victim for several weeks and mention drugs can shorten this span to a good extent. Tetanus immune globulin can be administered too for obtaining passive immunization for the victim up to few months. Pencillin IV is also to be administered to these victims for 2 weeks along with tetanus toxoid.

**Tetanus Immune Globulin:** This an injectable solution made of globulin of an immune. This is much safer and effective than the tetanus antitoxin. This will help into a short term vaccine for tetanus and it is always a part of tetanus treatment.

**Throat Culture:** This is a test conducted to throat to find out the organism that is posing into the disease for the victim throat. Specimen from the throat will be collected for this test with the help of long-handles sterile swab. This specimen will be tested culture plate and study will be conducted for 48 hours.

**Tinea:** This is fungal infection to the skin, nails and hair. This infection is caused through a fungi group known as dermatophytes and these are also known as ringworms too. The fungus species reason for this infection is epidemophyton, microsporum and trichophyton. Symptoms of this infection will vary basing on the affected portion of the body and foot is a very common prey for this disease. There will be cracking, itchy sensation between toes, and some more. Antifungal drugs are right choice to treat effectively this disease. Widespread disease will require this antifungal drug in the form of a tablet. It is essential to continue the treatment for few days after the symptoms were successfully faded out too. A simple mild infection will require six weeks treatment.

**Tinea Barbae:** This is ringworm infection to skin happens underneath beard through tinea mentagrophytes or through T. verrucosum.

**Tinea Capitis:** This is a medical term used for the scalp ringworm.

**Tinea Corporis:** This is the medical term for the very well-known body ringworm.

**Tinea Cruris:** This is jock itch and medical terms called as tinea cruris.

**Tinea Manuum:** This is another type of ringworm infection causes through tinea rubrum and it is foot infection. Treatment for this infection is antifungals along with oral antifungal drug like ketoconazole or griseofulvin or terbinafine. Treatment should be continued up to 3 mnths.

**Tinea Nigrapalmaris:** This is another type of superficial skin ringworm infection happens to the palms and sole of feet. This may look like malignant, but not a serious infection. Symptoms will be brown-black macule along with defined margins and seen spreading in circular forms. Treatment for this infection would be imidazole cream and use some scraping removal too like emery pad.

**Tinea Versicolor:** This is fungal skin infection called as pityriasis versicolor too. The fungus reason for this infection lives like a yeast on human skin and known as malassezia furfur. The symptoms are pale and tan patches over upper arms and upper trunk with itch. There is a chance for lesions with dark-skinned people. This disease is identified through the patches and treatment is antifungal cream application.

**Toe Web Infection:** This is a disorder of space between toes and called as athlete's foot too. This is a fungla infection causes through tissue destruction. There are more types of organisms are involved in this disease and this will require usage of several treatment options for the effective results. For lesions scaly and dry can use miconazole or ciclopirox olamine or clotrimazole. For lesions wet and soft can use daily compress along with tropical antimicrobial agent.

**Tonsillitis:** This tonsillitis are great help to stop infection and safeguard upper respiratory. Here, it is quite imperative to mention that the tonsillitis infected quite easily on own. The symptoms will be sore throat, headache, fever, ear ache, problem with swallowing, and tender lymph nodes. Acute condition can lead into Scarlet fever too. Tonsillitis treated successfully with the help of systematic antibiotics. Surgical procedure is nowadays not essential as antibiotics are successful to treat this problem.

**Tonsils:** These tonsils are formed as mass oval lymphoid on either side to moth back. This is a perfect defense system against the infections. These tonsils will turn into bigger down the line up to age seven and they will shrink on own subsequently. If these tonsils are infected, then it will leads to tonsillitis.

**Toxic Shock Syndrome:** This is severe skin rash condition that is quite uncommon and resemble almost like sun burn over soles and palms. This type of condition is caused through toxin produced through staphylococcus aureus known as enterotoxin. F. Symptoms will be high fever, diarrhea, vomiting, dizziness, muscular pain, headache and disorientation. There is a chance for 3% of severe cases to turn into deaths. Antibiotics along with IV fluids are the required treatment for this disease. Women suffering from toxic shock should keep away from using tampons, diaphragms, vaginal contraceptives, and cervical caps.

**Toxocara Canis:** This is a type of roundworm found mostly in dogs. This T. catis is less infectious than infestation called as toxocariasis.

**Toxocariasis:** This is an infection causes through the larvae of the toxocara cariis roundworm. These larvae often seen in soil and reaches into the human body through various possible choices. There is a long incubation period with this infection. Children infected through large numbers of larvae will be sick through breathing problems, pneumonia, liver enlargement, anemia, fever, skin rash, and fatigue and eye problems. This infection is diagnosed through the abnormal blood count that is with high number antibodies and a type of white blood cells. There is a no specific treatment for this problem or to cure infestation. This is a self-limiting disease leaves without treatment.

**Toxoid:** This is a bacterial toxin can be treated successfully with chemicals or through heat for reducing the toxic effect.

**Toxoplasma:** this is a crescent shaped parasite lives successfully within cells of various types of tissues and in organs of the vertebrate animals.

**Toxoplasmosis:** This is a disease happens through parasite called as toxoplasma gondii and it will be transmitted successfully to humans through contaminated soil, undercooked meat, or through direct contact from an infected individual. Cat very much involved in the transmission process as parasite excretes egg into cat's feces and from there it reaches animals and humans successfully. Symptoms will be mild through swelling lymph nodes at different places in the body along with fever, sore throat, tiredness and body rash. Blood test is essential part of diagnosis of this disease. Severe disease condition can be treated successfully with sulfonamides or with pyrimethamine. Healthy individuals and pregnant women will not require any treatment procedure.

**Trachoma:** This is a chronic infectious disease to eye happen through chlamydia trachomatis bacteria. This disease is more often to be seen with children and their mothers. This disease is easy to transmit through unclean water and through flies. Symptoms will be severe inflammation and pain to eye due to the light. Here is a chance to form thick scar tissue over upper eye lid, when untreated. This will turn into bigger lumps to cause into cornea damage and eventual blindness. It is highly important to treat this disease during early stage. Doctors will eradicate organism completely that is causing trachoma and doctors will administer drug directly into the eye for the people that sensitive to antibiotics.

**Traveler's Diarrhea:** This traveler's diarrhea is a common disease to people that is frequently traveled to tropics. This disease is caused through intestinal bacteria known as escherichia coli. Symptoms will be diarrhea, bloating, nausea and malaise. Symptoms will be there up to one week. There is no treatment for disease and it will subside on own.

**Treponema:** This is a genus belongs to the spirochetes and these are reasons for the syphilis, pinta and yaws for humans.

**Treponema Pallidum:** this is one of the active spirochete to cause syphilis.

**Trichinella Spiralis:** This is roundworm in intestinal and causes trichinosis.

**Trichinosis:** This is another food-borne disease through microscopic intestinal roundworm known as trichinella spiralis. These worm larvae generally reside within infested animal muscles as cyst. This will transmit to human through uncooked meat or raw meat. This will be active within six weeks after eating the uncooked meat by the victim. Symptoms will be purely based on incubation period and this is again dependent over the worm burden. Infestation happened through less volume of worms will not show any kind of symptoms over the victim. Symptoms in general will be diarrhea along with fever, vomiting, pneumonia, respiratory failure and heart failure. Symptoms are the only possible choice to diagnosis this disease and it can also be confirmed through blood test too. Treatment for this disease will be thiabendazole, cortisteroids and painkillers. Bed rest is highly essential for these victims as there is a chance for the death too through this disease. Total treatment can take up to three months duration.

**Trichomonas Vaginalis:** This is a protozoan with single and capable enough to cause vaginal infection.

**Trichomoniasis:** This is an infection to vagina through protozoan and it is a STD. There is a chance for this disease to transmit through washcloth or baby or through towel of the infected female too. There is a chance for this infection in male too that are with infected urethra. The protozoan called as trichomonas vaginalis is the reason for this disease. Symptoms will be inflammation with pain, vaginal itching, smelly discharge, and painful sex. Vaginal discharge in lab can detect this disease successfully. Treatment is through metronidazole and this medication should be considered for infected and partner too.

**Trichosporosis:** This is a fungus condition happens to hair through hard masses fungus in the color of black or white. It is essential to remove infected hair through shaving as a best treatment option.

**Tropical Disease:** Temperate areas are prone to diseases and these are widespread only in tropics and some other infectious diseases are confined within the tropical areas. Pverty, temperature conditions, disease carry insects, humidity are always prevalent in this particular part of world. Malnutrition is another major reason for the growth of infectious diseases in tropics.

**Trypanosomiasis:** This is another tropical disease happens through parasitic protozoa known as trypanosomes. The African tryponosomiasis infection generally transmitted through testes fly bite to humans. Symptoms will be skin inflammation, fever, and rash, pain to skin, enlarged lymph nodes and anemia. This disease requires immediate treatment unless will turn into quite fatal. Toxic drugs are ideal to treat this disease and these drugs should be used with utmost precaution. Early stage treatment can bring good results over the victim. There is a chance for death or irreversible brain damage, when not treated this disease.

**Tuberculin Test:** This is a skin test performed to find out the tuberculosis for a person.

**Tuberculosis:** this is a respiratory disease spreads very fast from person to person via air. This TB is caused through three different species of mycrobacteria known as M. africanuum, M.bovis and Mycobacterium tuberculosis. Symptoms will be chest pain or cough, which can stay up to 2 weeks. Later stage victim will start to cough up blood or sometimes with phlegm from lungs. Victim will turn into weak with loss of appetite, weight loss, fever and chills. This disease can be diagnosed only through tuberculin skin test. Patient should be isolated as a part of the treatment and tested regularly. Nowadays, there are wide varieties of drugs are available to treat TB effectively unlike olden days. It is completely curable and patient will not be infectious after the successful treatment.

**Tuberculosis, Skin:** This is an infection causes through direct inoculation of mycobacteriun tuberculosis into the victim wound. There will be inflammatory nodule through this disease and this is called as tuberculoous chancre. There will be lymph nodes inflammation along with vessels. Treatment for this disease is through antituberculosis drugs up to one year.

**Tularemia:** This is an infectious disease for animals and often seen infected to humans too. This disease is caused through francisella (Pasteurella0 tualrensis bacteria, which enters into the body through a scratch or cut over the skin. This disease also transmitted through bite of a tick or flea or fly or louse or through consuming infected rabbit meat. Symptoms will be skin lesion, enlarged lymph nodes, fever, chills, muscle pain, headache, malaise and fatigue. Antibiotics like tetracycline and streptomycin are ideal treatment for this disease.

**Tungiasis:** this is a skin infection happens through flea burrowing, Symptoms of this disease are localized rash to skin along with lesions that are with live fleas. Treatment for this infection will be ideal through ethyl chloride spray and apply it all over the lesions.

**Typhoid Fever:** This is a serious and fatal bacterial infection to the intestinal tract. This typhoid fever happens through slamonella typhi bacteria. The bacteria initially reside within intestine and multiples to invade the blood stream of the patient. Symptoms will be fever, joint pains, headache, constipation and sore throat. This disease is diagnosed through culture test and from blood sample. Antibiotics are successful to shorten the problem and reduce complications too to a great extent.

**Typhus:** This typhus is caused through rickettsiae and transmitted through lice that are from the infected patients' blood. These lice will leave the feces over other people skin to result into infection. Symptoms are measles kind rash, headache, limb pain, high fever, weak heartbeat, confusion, delirium and prostration. This disease can be diagnosed successfully with the help of checking blood for the rickettsia organisms. Antibiotics can treat typhus more effectively and some more medications can be sought to obtain relief from symptoms.

**Typhus, Endemic Flea-Borne:** This endemic flea typhus disease is generally transmitted to humans through infected rat flea bite. Symptoms will be fever and rash over trunk and these symptoms will stay up to 2 weeks, Antibiotics are available to treat this disease effectively. This is a not a fatal problem.

**Typhus, Epidemic Louse-Borne:** This is a parasite caused infection causes through transmission from infected person to other due to lice infestation. Symptoms will be headache, chills and pains. Drug therapy is a right choice to treat this disease effectively. Isolation is essential for the patient until entire lice eliminated from the patient.

**Typhus, Scrub:** This is a disease through mite also called as tsutsugamushi too. This disease generally transmitted through the infected rodents and parasites via mites. Symptoms will be backache and headache. There is a chance for swelling at the mite-bite spot, which turns into blisters down the line. There is a treatment procedure available from physician to treat this problem more effectively.

**Infectious Diseases Start with "U"**

**Universal Precautions:** This is an approach to control infections and to prevent transmission of the all types of blood-borne diseases like Hepatitis B and AIDS Through proper health care setting. These precautions were initially designed by U.S. Centers for Disease Control in the year 1987 and also created by the Bureau of Communicable Disease Epidemiology in Canada in the year of 1989.

**Urethritis:** This is an infection, which can cause inflammation to the urethra and this disease generally causes through organisms that are common cause for gonorrhea too. Here, nonspecific urethritis will happen through different varieties microorganisms and bacteria like chlamydia or yeasts. This bacterium is capable enough to spared to rectum or skin from urethra too. Symptoms will be pain along with burning feeling while urinating and it can turn into quite severe too. Sometimes, there will be strains of blood through urine too. If this is caused due to gonorrhea, then there will be yellow color pus-filled discharge. Treatment is considered for the underlying infection, when infected with urethritis. Gonorrhea can be easily treated with antibiotics or Pencillin. Treatment for nonspecific urethritis will dependent over the caused organism and treatment should be decided basing on it.

**Urinary Tract Infection (UTI):** This is also called as bladder infection too and it is a bacterial infection. This UTI is caused through bacteria that are originated from vagina or rectum. Symptoms will be urging for frequent urination and pain during urination. This disease diagnosis in lab is conducted through urinalysis and urine will be cultured for 48 hours for this test. Treatment for this disease is more effective through wide varieties of antibacterial drugs along with flushing the bladder with plenty of fluids.

## Infectious Diseases Start with "V"

**Vaccine:** Vaccine is a tiny dosage of a particular protein belongs to the organism that is causing disease. This will prevent the disease successfully. Vaccine will help to develop protection to the body against invasion through disease causing organisms. There are many types of vaccines available and those are Anthrax, pneumonia, diphtheria, chicken pox, German measles, influenza, Hepatitis B, Hepatitis A, Lyme disease, Mumps, malaria, plague, whooping cough, Q fever, polio, tetanus, rabies, tuberculosis, small pox, yellow fever and typhoid.

**Vaginal Infection:** This infection generally causes through yeast or bacteria. Diagnosis of vaginal infection requires examination of vaginal fluids through microscope. Some types of vaginal infection will cause through vaginitis and symptoms will be irritation, itching and discharge.

**Vaginal Yeast Infection:** This infection is also called as candidiasis too. This infection causes through yeast that is normally found within vagina. This vaginal infection will happen through upsetting of delicate balance like obesity, diabetes, pregnancy, steroids usage and some more. Symptoms will be thick and white discharge along with itching. There is a chance for swelling to vagina or vulva too. Vaginal culture is the right diagnosis procedure to find out this disease. There are few over the counter drugs available to treat this infection in the form of suppositories and creams.

**Vaginitis (vaginosis):** This is a mild infection to vagina and sometimes inflammation to vagina can also be considered vaginitis. This infection causes through gardnerella vaginalis bacteria. The symptoms will be vaginal discharge frothy or sometimes in gray in color. There will be bad odor too with this discharge. Besides discharge, there will be itching, irritation and burning too. Treatment for this vaginosis will be antibiotics like metronidazole, but this drug is prohibited from using for the female during their initial 14 weeks pregnancy.

**Valley Fever:** This is also known as cocci or coccidioidomycosis.

**Vancomycin-Resistant Enterococci:** This is a bacterium commonly infects patients that are in the intensive-care. These bacteria are quite resistant to antibiotics and this is causing into huge threat for the public-health.

**Varicella-Zoster Immune Globulin (VZIG):** The immune globulin is generally sought from normal people blood that is with highest levels of varicella-zoster-antibodies. This immune globulin is generally used as a treatment for chicken pox, which is capable enough to prevent as well as reduces the symptoms too.

**Varicella-Zoster Virus (VZV):** This is a virus belongs to the family of herpes virus and causes varicella disease and herpes zoster. This is a highly contagious virus and capable enough to spread through direct contact or through droplets.

**Venereal Diseases:** Sexually transmitted diseases are also called as venereal diseases.

**Vibrio:** This is a type of bacterium in curved shape with a capacity to unconscious movement and tail makes them the best swimmers. The bacteria that belong to this category are V. cholerae, vibrio parahaemolyticus, V. alginolticus and V. vulnificus. There are some more marine vibrios are present in the environment to cause into several diseases for humans.

**Vibrio Cholerae:** This is bacteria in the shape of comma and it will cause cholera to humans.

**Vibrio Parahamolyticus:** This is a type of bacterium that is originated from sea fish and shell fish to cause food poisoning.

**Vibrios Parahaemolyticus Gastroenteritis:** This is a type of blood poisoning disease happens through eating a variety of fish or contaminated shellfish. Generally, this disease route cause is V. parahaemolyticus bacteria that is lives within shellfish or some other type of sea fish. Symptoms will be seen within 4 days and there will be diarrhea, nausea, vomiting and abdominal cramps. This disease can be diagnosed through the stool culture in the lab. Treatment for this disease will be purely symptomatic along with clear fluids. Generally, this infection tend to clear up within a short span of time on own.

**Vincent's Disease:** This disease is also called as trench mouth and it is a bacterial infection. This disease is caused through microorganisms, which are harmless and seen within the pockets of gums. Some of the reasons for this infection are smoking, inappropriate dental hygiene, throat infection, impaired or weak immune system and emotional stress. Symptoms will sore gums along with bleeding and ulcers will be found over gums with bleeding. There will be bad breathe too along with glands swelling. Treatment for this disease will be mouthwash that is with hydrogen peroxide. Some of the proven antibacterial drugs can also result into a good treatment for this problem.

**Viral infection:** These are common infectious diseases caused through virus. Viral infections are generally mild and sometimes can be more dangerous too. Mild viral infections are common cold and warts. The severe viral infections are rabies, small pox, AIDS, and poliomyelitis.

**Virucide:** This is an agent that is capable enough to destroy virus.

**Virus:** This is a tiny infectious agent and a parasitic organism. These are very small than bacteria with no independent metabolic activity.

**Vulvovaginitis:** This is an infection to vulva and vagina through trichomoniasis or through candidiasis. This is a yeast infection results into inflammation for vagina and vulva. There will be intense vaginal discharge due to this infection. Treatment will be effective for this disease through antibiotics or antifungal drugs.

## Infectious Diseases Start with "W"

**Warts:** These are harmless tiny round bumps along with rough surface and happen generally over hands, knees, fingers and genitals. The common type of warts is digitate warts, filiform warts, flat warts, plantar warts, and some more. These warts will happen through more than 58 types of human papillomavirus (HPV). Most of the warts are contagious and spreads through personal contact quite easily. Most types of warts diagnosis will be made through their appearance and rarely require biopsy. Treatment for warts has no specific treatment as more than 65% of warts disappear automatically within a certain span of time. There are few over the counter drugs are available to treat warts in the form of tropical medication with salicylic acid and some more ointments.

**Warts, Genital:** These are soft warts normally appear at the entry of vagina, anus and the penis. These genital warts come under the STD category. These genital warts will cause through 8 different varieties of human papillomavirus. These warts will be in the color of pink or grey with soft raised surface with itching and burning. There will be bleeding to around genital due to these warts. Diagnosis of the warts and their condition will be done through doctor basing on their appearance with the help of magnifying glass. There is no specific treatment for these warts and eradication of traces is hard to accomplish. Treatment is always aimed towards elimination of warts shrinking with the help of tropical solution or through laser or through surgery. There is a huge chance for the reappearance of warts after the treatment too.

**Water, Contaminated:** Very often, water is the major source for the contamination and infection and water contains many types of parasitic or infective organisms. Tainted water is always being a great source throughout the world for spreading all types of infectious diseases.

**Waterhouse-Friderichsen Syndrome:** This is a serious and rare infection causes through meningococcus group bacteria. Symptoms will be coma for the victim within hours due to the blood pouring into the adrenal glands. This wil lead to acute adrenal failure too. Treatment for this disease is always through emergency treatment procedure and with vasopressor drugs. Treatment should include intravenous fluids, oxygen and plasma.

**Weil's Syndrome:** This is a severe condition of leptospirosis and this infectious disease causes through leptospira genus organisms. These organisms will be transmitted through urine of domestic and wild animals. Symptoms will be kidney and liver problems along with meningitis and vomiting. Antibiotics are the choicest treatment facility for this disease.

**Whipple's Disease:** This is a very rare type of intestinal disorder happens through abnormal skin pigmentation. This disease generally happens to mid-age male. The root cause of this disease is still unknown, but probably due to bacterial infection. Symptoms will be malabsorption, abdominal pain, and diarrhea, wright loss, swelling to lymph nodes, joint pains, fever and anemia. Jejunal biopsy is needed to diagnosis this disease. Antibiotics like Pencillin or tetracycline can be effective treatment for this disease.

**Whipworm Infestation (Trichuriasis):** Whipworms are roundworms and parasites. These roundworms belong to the trichuris trichura species, which can infect intestinal tract of the human. This whipworm infection transmitted through personal contact and eggs of this worm will be hatched and embedded within the mucous membranes. Symptoms will be bloody diarrhea, when worm burden is huge. Stool examination is the suitable diagnosis procedure to identify this infection. Treatment for this infection is ideal through mebendazole and this drug capable enough to kill the worms successfully.

**Whitmore's Disease:** This disease is also called as melioidosis and it is totally an uncommon variety bacterial infection. This disease will also be seen in animals like pigs, sheep, cattle and horses. The exact disease transmission is quite clueless, but causes through breathing bacteria that is emitted from broken skin. Symptoms will be may appear within a month and above years due to the exact incubation period is still unknown. There will be acute blood poisoning and diarrhea through this disease. Treatment for this disease will be antibiotics and abscesses should be eliminated through surgery.

**Whooping Cough:** This whooping cough is also called as pertussis too and it is an acute infection to the upper respiratory tract. This disease generally spreads through cough of the infected individual. The bacteria are capable enough to survive over bed covers, tissue for short duration. This disease can be easily transmitted from the infected individual to other family members. Symptoms will be cold like conditions along with sneezing, sore eyes and low-fever. There will be irritating dry cough for a period of 2 weeks and this dry cough period will be totally infectious. Diagnosis of this disease will be through identifying the bacteria in culture that is grown from nasal swab. Early stage treatment is always ideal with this disease. Antibiotics like clarithromycin or erythromycin can offer good relief from the disease.

**World Health Organization:** This is an agency belongs to United Nations and established in the year of 1948. This agency will look after the international health concerns and public health. Geneva is the headquarters of this agency.

## Infectious Diseases Start with "Y"

**Yaws:** This is an infection and childhood skin problem too. This yaws is caused through spirochete treponema pertenue bacteria, which is belongs to T. palladium family. The symptoms will be malaise, headache and low fever. This is no fatal infection, but highly contagious. Site of the infection can be seen with red-itchy growth. Treatment will be single dosage of pencillin and it can heal on own too, but will take up to six months of time.

**Yeast Infection:** This is a type of skin infection happens through fungi known as candida albicans. This is a friendly fungi and normally seen in mouth, large intestine and in vagina. It will turn against to host, when consumed oral steroids or antibiotics or birth control drugs.

**Yellow Fever:** This is a short-acting viral infection and seen in the form of yellow colored skin as with jaundice. This yellow fever can be seen in three forms as urban, sylvan and jungle. This yellow fever causes through flavivirus and flavus means yellow in Latin. Most of the yellow fever cases will not show any symptoms. Some will have mild illness and this illness can lead to death too. People with symptoms will have sudden fever within 6 days along with headache, nausea, backache, and vomiting. Urine test results with huge levels of albumin or blood test results with low count of white blood cells will prove this disease presence in victim. Drugs are not effective against this disease and treatment will always aim to offer relief from symptoms.

**Yersinia Enterocolitica:** This is a tiny bacteria belong to Yersinia genus and causes entercolitis.

**Yersinia (pasteurella) Pestis:** This is a tiny gram negative bacterium to cause plague in humans and transmits this disease through rodents or flea.

**Yersinia Psudotuberculosis:** These bacteria belong to Yersinia genus and causes pseudotuberculosis to humans.

**Yersiniosis:** This is a food-borne disease caused through consuming tainted food or through direct contact from sick pets or contaminated individuals. Two varieties of species bacteria reason for this disease and those are Yersinia pseudotuberculosis and yersinia anterocolitica. Symptoms will be high fever along with vomiting, nausea, diarrhea, pain in abdomen and some more. Stool culture can be a suitable diagnosis procedure to identify this disease. Antibiotics are the best treatment option for this disease and serious cases will deserve hospitalization along with intravenous medication.

## VOLUME II

Many reports are currently indicating that STD is high relatively within the Thailand. One of the surveys recently indicated that this STD seen with 49% male and 11% female in urban areas. The most common forms of STD are non-gonococcal urethritis and gonorrhea, which is seen in male and urethritis and chlamydia that are seen in female. The rate of occurrence of this STD is high within the Thailand due to the improper awareness towards the issue and its prevention measures. Most of the victims are seen belongs to the lower socio-economic group people. Here, it is quite imperative to mention that the HIV and AIDS relatively and to a great extent associated with few STD infections like gonorrhea, syphilis, genital warts, genital herpes and few more.

Most of the STD disease infections within the Thailand can be successfully attributed to the commercial sex market. Many past reports at this place indicated that the 95% infected male admitting with clinics their past sexual encounters with commercial sex services. Government STD clinics in Thailand witnessing this issue seriously and addressing it through offering free treatment services and regular examinations for the public and sex workers on regular basis. They suggest and encourage victims of STD and sex workers to visit their clinics once in a week without fail to have regular checkups and examinations. Government initiated sincere surveillance against the source of the STD infections and considering reports of the victims about the source of infection too. This is enabling government STD clinics to initiate necessary examinations and treatments for the sex workers located in that particularly mentioned source.

This kind of action is resulting into an effective precautionary measure against the STD and its control.

**Non-Specific Urethritis**

Inflammation to urethra is known as Urethritis and this is a tube, where urine for the human passes. There are so many reasons to list for the urethra inflammation and this is making this issue as non-specific urethritis.

Infection is not necessarily being the main reason for the urethra inflammation. There is a chance for this inflammation through physical irritation too. This physical irritation generally happens through damaged lining, which can result into discharge too. Also, there is a strong chance for this inflammation through the strong substance too.

Signs and Symptoms

Inflammation can happen through many types of infections for a human. It can be categorized into two categories basing on the current available treatment procedures. The category one is known as gonococcal urethritis that is generated through the gonorrhea infection. The category two is known as non-gonococcal urethritis that is generated through the chlamydial infection. There are some more inflammations to generate through the ureaplasma and mycoplasma too. In some of the very rare cases, Herpes can result into inflammation too. The inflammation with both categories having more chances to subside within two days, but root caused infection should be treated effectively.

Treatments

The main characteristic of the urethritis is severe pain that associates well with genital discharge.

Treatment for this issue should be initiated purely basing on the root cause, which is already mentioned above. Non-specific urethritis treatment will be easy through common prescription medication, which is generated basing on the root causes of gonorrhea and chlamydia. The mentioned root causes are easy to treat through proper and suitable drugs.

- Azithromycin (Azith, Zithromax) 1 g orally in a single dose
- Doxycycline (Vibramycin) 100 mg orally twice a day for 7 days
- Ofloxacin (Tarivid, Floxin) 300 mg orally twice a day for 7 days

Antibiotic treatment is suitable for this issue, when there is no traces infection for the individual.

Genital warts are generally developed through the HPV or human papilloma virus and these warts are also known as condylomata acuminta or venereal warts or cauliflower disease too. This issue generally starts to develop in male and female at anal and genital region in the form of cauliflower shape warts or gray-colored warts or flesh warts. There is a chance to witness this issue within throat or mouth of the infected individual too.

These genital warts are more contagious with a more than 60% of chances for acquisition with single sex contact, and this is a top most commonly seen STD through a dangerous virus. In Thailand, more than 70% of the female sex workers got this disease and 20% among them got other STD issues along with the mentioned genital warts.


Causes

The main reason for the genital warts is HPV or human papilloma virus. There are more than 10 varieties of HPV identified so far and 40 varieties among them will have more chances to infect human genital areas. There are two specific HPV verities namely HPV-6 and HPV-11 commonly found over 90% genital warts issues. Luckily, these two varieties are with very less potential to result the issue into cancer.

There is a latency period for this virus once after penetrated successfully into the human skin. There is a chance for some people to experience warts within 3 month duration and some fail to experience any signs of it too. The symptoms will stay for a period of two month to years in few cases. This is very popular through its contagious nature and disease passes successfully from one to other without any slightest knowledge.

Signs and Symptoms

The issue genital warts are totally painless. There is a chance for uncomfortable conditions for the individual through the developed warts through itching and irritation. Sometimes, this uncomfortable condition will be added up with discharge too. The size of the warts will always vary in different ways with a chance for joining together too. These warts in male can be seen developing over rectal location, penis and scrotum. In female, it will appear in most locations such as vagina opening and some more. Sometimes lesions are seen developing across outer genital areas too. There is a chance for urine obstruction or bleeding, when wart grown over urethral opening area.

Diagnosis

An individual should inform doctor about the complete history of the wart from the day of its appearance over the body. There is a special technique normally used to view the lesions with more clarity through using aceto-whitening. Acetic acid will be applied all over the affected portion to view the lesion completely well in this technique. This acid solution usage will turn the affected area into white within ten minutes after the application. A Pap smear test or some other lab test can be considered to find out the presence of the HPV infection for an individual.

Treatment

Genital warts can be treated successfully with many varieties of options. Here, any of the treatment procedure is failing to control the comeback of the warts successfully. Treatments are successful to get rid of the wart, but fail to eliminate HPV completely well. It is highly tough or not possible to eliminate this infection once after it start to present in the individual's body.

Some popular treatments for genital warts in Thailand include:

Podophyllotoxin Paint (Condylline)- Apply this all over the affected portion weekly basis and leave the affected area for one to six hours before washing it off. Daily, it is suggested applying 0.5% of alcoholic gel or 0.15% of cream for total three days without washing the affected portion. Repeat this procedure for totally 5 weeks. It is good to stop this treatment after five weeks, when there is no expected result.

Imiquimod 5% Cream (Aldara) - Apply this cream all over the affected area and leave it for six to ten hours before washing. This should be practiced three times in a week for alternate nights. Try this treatment for sixteen weeks duration and stop the treatment, when there is no reasonable relief after 16 weeks through this treatment.

Cryotherapy- This is liquid nitrogen, which is to be applied all over the warts to freeze them and this should be practiced once in a week. Few weeks of this treatment can help well to clear off the warts successfully.

Laser treatment is another wise option for the places of the body that are highly tough to reach and treat with alternate methods. Also, this laser treatment is an option, where issues are quite resistant with other treatment procedures too.

Prevention

An HPV Vaccine (Gardasil, Cervarix) is the best wise choice for male and female as early as 9 years old for the perfect protection against certain varieties of HPV.

**Herpes:**

Herpes is another dangerous and more contagious disease happens through the herpes simplex virus. There is around 70% sex workers in Thailand infected with this disease according to the latest reports. This is currently rampant all over Thailand due to the lack of awareness about its quick transmission among people. The current victims are result through the failure of identifying symptoms, or not diagnosing the issue in time, or sometimes herpes fails to show significant signs for a longer duration too. The genital herpes can result into lesions and blisters all around the genital area both in male and female.

Causes

This herpes simplex virus, which is reason for herpes can be seen in two common varieties. The HSV 1 is very usual virus to result into blisters and lesions all over the lips, face and mouth. This can transmit quite quickly through kiss or genital or oral contact. The HSV 2 can result into genital herpes infections for people. This virus happens in general between two people, but there is a huge chance to spread through skin to skin contact too.

This virus generally gets entry through skin and settles successfully and permanently near to the spine area. Initially, it will stay calm with no symptoms or signs for years. The infection resulted through this virus is permanent and treatment procedures will help to eliminate the blisters and lesions alone and not the infection.

Signs and Symptoms

This infection generally starts to show its impact through blisters and typical redness. The outbreak is little slower and takes years to show severe impact. The lesions resulted through this infection will be almost like open sores all over the affected portion of the body. Very commonly, these symptoms can be seen developing at the mouth corners or all across genital area basing on the type of infection.

This virus is inactive for many years since after settling within the spinal cord of the individual and this will create complete unaware conditions about the issue for a longer period. There is a chance to experience symptoms with the virus at the earliest within two weeks and sometimes it may take years too. Sometimes, there will be no symptoms at all too. The outbreak will reoccur again and again after treating the blisters and lesions with suitable treatment procedures. The healing period for lesions and blisters is generally three weeks. In some cases, this infection can leave no traces of symptoms too.

Diagnosis

Clinical examination can reveal the presence of HSV-1 successfully. This will be easy to identify within the individual, when there is no prior history of blisters or lesions and came in contact with someone that is already infected with HSV-1. The diagnosis of the HSV-2 is little difficult as this is not well associated with any classical symptoms. There is a chance to be mistaken with other issue that is with similar symptoms too. Laboratory testing is the only left out option for this purpose. You can consider wide varieties of tests for this purpose such as blood test, direct fluorescent antibody study, skin biopsy, virus culture, polymerase test, viral DNA some more.

Treatment

The infection with this issue is always permanent and treatment procedures cannot eradicate the virus permanently. The herpes is generally harmless, but lesions resulted will show their impact with inflammation, irritation and uncomfortable conditions. Prescription drugs for this infection can offer reasonable relief against resulted symptoms and controls the outbreak to a great extent.

- Acyclovir (Acivir, Vilerm) 400mg given orally twice a day for 5-7 days

- Valacyclovir (Valtrex) 500 mg orally twice a day for 5-10 days

- Famciclovir (Famvir) 250 mg three times a day for 5 days

.

Acyclovir Cream (Acivir, Vilerm)- Apply this cream five times in a day with hourly intervals for a period of five to ten days.

There are few proven alternative medicines and dietary supplements for treating this issue. These are widely popular all over Thailand such as antioxidant therapy and special herbal drugs. The effective treatment against to the infection through these alternate medicines is currently got no scaffolding evidence to prove benefits. In fact, these special treatments are ideal to improve immune system and this will control recurrence of the outbreak to a great extent.

**Syphilis:**

Syphilis is another infection resulted through the microscopic bacterial organisms known as spirochete bacterium. A microscope can offer the look of this bacterial organism as spiral shape worm which wiggles constantly. This bacterium occupies moist and mucous-covered lining area of the mouth upon transmission. This bacterium starts producing painless ulcer in the form of chancre.

Signs and Symptoms

The common symptoms associated with syphilis are categorized into four different stages, which include a latent stage.

Primary stage of syphilis can be seen in the form of single pain free non-itchy sore and this can occupy over genital area according to the chances. Generally, this will be transmitted through a person that is already infected with this infection. It takes ten day to sixteen weeks period after the successful transmission to present chancre. There is a chance to develop multiple lesions in some cases too. It is highly imperative to realize that these lesions are very contagious. These lesions can appear for weeks to a month and disappears automatically without any treatment. But, treatment is essential keeping in mind its recurrence into the secondary stage of the syphilis.

The secondary stage of syphilis will start to appear after the four to ten weeks after the first stage of the infection. The chancre spots and lesions will start to reappear again with symmetrical form reddish pink rashes with no itchy feeling. These rashes will appear over trunk, feet, hands and extremities. Slowly, these will transform into wart kind of lesions. These lesions are dangerous and successful to harbor bacteria too. There will be some more added symptoms to this stage with fever, sore throat, body malaise, hair loss and headache.

There is a chance for no symptoms with some individuals with this secondary stage of syphilis too. This kind of phase is widely called as latent phase. Generally, this phase will endure for few months to years too.

Tertiary syphilis is next stage to happen, which will emerge within three to fifteen years of the secondary stage of the infection. There is a chance for relapses with the second stage symptoms, but infection will be widespread for sure. This stage of infection will have chances to affect the body internal organs and mainly impacts badly over nervous system, brain and heart. Insanity is another important symptom occurs with this stage of infection. Failing to treat this stage will result into disabilities and death for the victim.

The last stage of the infection fails to show any symptoms over the victim. This stage will take the syphilis to maximum extent to result into ravage over the body. Infection will be widespread in this stage. Syphilis will start to attack internal organs rampant over bones, heart, nervous system and brain. This stage deserves effective treatment as the life will be at the stake when failed to treat properly.

Diagnosis

It is highly tough to diagnose syphilis in early days of the infection. It should be predicted basing upon the chancre appearance. A blood test will be reasonable help to confirm the infection. There will be follow-up tests for the patient after the antibiotic treatment for a period of six months and these tests only can confirm the complete eradication of the infection.

Treatment

Treatment for syphilis should be considered basing up on its stage and this can be ascertained through the clinical manifestation.

For early manifestations, it is essential to have single dose of intramuscular penicillin G or single dose of oral azithromycin. If a person is allergic to penicillin, then ceftriaxone single IM dose of 250 mg may be ideal choice or penicillin desensitization attempted. Other alternative treatments include:

- Doxycycline 200 to 400 mg/day in divided doses orally for 10-15 days

- Tetracycline 200 to 400 mg/day in divided doses orally for 10-15 days

The treatment of neurosyphilis requires the intravenous administration of penicillin

## Molluscum Contagiosum:

Molluscum contagiosum (MC) is widely known as "the calm" all over the Thailand. It is a viral skin infection seen in the form of tiny, firm spots erupted over the skin to transform into clustered lesions. These are totally free from pain, but there is a chance for moderate itchy feeling according to few proven reports. This infection will start to disappear automatically, but resulted lesions will be definitely annoying and unattractive too. This infection is generally confines to mucous membranes and skin only. This infection will transmit to other through skin contact from an already infected individual. This infection is commonly seen all over the world and especially with children, immuno-deficient individuals and sexually active people. Currently, this infection is one of the rampant STDs in Thailand. Tropical climate and some other living conditions are also reasonable factors for this infection too.

Causes

The molluscum contagiosum virus is the major reason behind this infection and transmitted quite quickly through simple skin contact. The objects that are used by the infected individual will have more chances to transmit this disease with others and this is widely known as formites too. There are four different viruses for this infection as MCV- 1 to MCV-4. Here, the MCV-1 is quite prevalent and MCV-2 is generally seen with sexually active adults and transmission happens through sex. Currently, MCV-2 is quite rampant in the Thailand. The lesions will start to appear within two to seven weeks and stays up to duration of six months.

Signs and Symptoms

The lesions occurred through MCV will be smoother with dome-shape and color of the affected skin will be with opalescent. The lesions are totally free from pain, but annoy little with irritation and itchy feeling. There is a chance for the infection scarring through scratching a lesion, which can turn into eruption. The center acme portion of the lesion generally will carry virus and this can be seen as waxy and depressed. The average size of the lesion will be two to six millimeters, but mainly depends over the stage of lesion development. Generally, infection will be limited up to local area of the skin top layer, but often spreads up to the neighboring locations of the skin too. This kind of situation is very often happens with children and this is known as autoinoculation.

This virus very often shows its impact over the body trunk portion, legs and arms. The infection resulted through sex will affect badly over groin, thighs, lower abdomen and genital area.

Diagnosis

Clinical appearance is the best choice to diagnoses this infection within an individual. Virus culture is a not a wise option for this purpose and excisional biopsy is the wise choice.

Treatment

This Molluscum Contagiosum is totally a self-limited disease. Lesions developed through this infection will disappear automatically after two to three months duration. This virus should be controlled through medical treatment keeping in mind its autoinoculation condition. Treatment is unnecessary, but annoying irritation and itchy feelings will drive an individual to seek suitable medication. Here, treatment is nothing, but just traumatizing the lesion. There is a chance for scarring or pigmentary through this treatment.

Some treatments for MCV available in Thailand include:

Cryosurgery – Apply liquid nitrogen (dry ice) to each individual lesion. Repeat treatments in 2-3 weeks interval.

Podophyllotoxin – Apply 15% (Indian podophyllum) or up to 25% solution (American podophyllum) on the warts once a week. Leave for 1-6 hours and then wash it off. Stop the treatment if no improvement is observed after 6 weeks. Alternatively, apply 0.5% alcoholic gel or 0.15% cream two times a day for 3 days but do not wash it off. Repeat for up to 5 weeks.

Salicylic Acid – After cleaning the area, apply 60% solution directly then cover with plaster. Repeat the process until lesions become soft which will be about 3-7 days.

Imiquimod – As 5% cream, apply 3 times weekly for 4 weeks. The cream is applied at night and left on the skin for approximately 8 hours then wash off with mild soap and water. If no improvement is observed, a 4 week interval is needed before starting again on a 4 week treatment.

**Trichomoniasis:**

Trichomoniasis is another sexually transmitted disease seen very commonly in and around in the name of "trich'. The root cause for this disease is parasite and this will result into serious urogenital tract infection. This disease is more prone in female than male. Main reason for this phenomenon is that this trichomoniasis will stay asymptomatic in male and fails to record evidence and any other confirmation of its presence.

Causes

This trichomoniasis generally develops due to the parasite namely trichomonas vaginalis, which is a protozoan parasite. Generally, this parasite will pass from individual to other through and during intercourse. Size of this parasite is at an average of 15mm and its reproduction capabilities are huge with every eight to twelve hours. Still reasons are not found for this infection to happen more in female than male. In fact, both genders are purely susceptible to the infection. Treatment is essential for this infection as symptoms will result into health dangerous for both male and female, but there is a chance for male to expel the parasite within 14 days after the infection.

Signs and symptoms

It is characteristically observed that only women can experience symptoms associated with trichomoniasis. Some of the symptoms include vaginal discharge, vaginal itching. Inflammation of the cervix, urethra and vagina may also produce an itching and burning sensation. The vaginal discharge is usually yellow green, frothy and foul-smelling. In some cases, there is pain an urination and at the lower abdomen. For men, the parasite can become dormant for years. And since there is seldom any symptom, it can remain undetected. There are limited cases wherein men experience symptoms such as urethral discharge, a slight burning sensation after urination or ejaculation and pain and swelling of the scrotum.

Many research results observed symptoms experience only in female with trichomoniais. Most common symptoms associated with this disease are vagina itching, discharge from vagina, cervix inflammation, urethra and vagina itching, and itching sensation along with burning feel. The vaginal discharge resulted through this disease will normally be seen in yellowish green along with foul smell and froth. There is a chance for pain while urinating at lower abdomen area due to this infection. This parasite will be completely dormant in male for many years. This is causing failure to detection of infection in male too. There are few cases with male experiencing symptoms such as swelling along with pain of scrotum, urethra discharge, burning sensation during ejaculation and urination and some more.

Diagnosis

This trichomoniais diagnosis needs specimen from vagina that was collected from the pelvic examination. This sample will be observed through microscope in laboratory. This parasite will be generally identified from the sample in the shape of pear with too many of whip-like tails at one side of the end. This trichomoniasis cannot be found through the regular urine test, but presence of lesions and ulcerations is a perfect indication of this infection.

Treatment

It is highly necessary for both partners to consider treatment, when one sex partner identified with the trichomoniais disease. Metronidazole is the current standard treatment for this disease.

Metronidazole – A single dose of 2 grams for 2 days or 0.6 to 1 gram per day, three doses for 7 days. If symptoms persist, repeat medication after 4 to 6 week interval

Tenonitrozole – Take 250 mg twice a day for 4 days.


**Chlamydia:**

Chlamydia trachomatis is another common STD very often seen in the Thailand. In the year 2005, a Swedish government research and analysis firm mentioned that the Thailand as the one of the major sources for chlamydia infections. Current statics in Thailand indicating significant fall with this disease victims in Thailand as Spain is leading at top keeping Thailand next to it. Here, it is still an acceptable fact that chlamydia still exist within the Thailand.

Causes

This chlamydia is caused in humans due to the chlamydia trachomatis bacterium. This bacterium is capable enough to damage female reproductive organ directly. There are no obvious signs and symptoms associated with this disease and this is creating a great chance to miss or ignore these symptoms in a female. Treatment for this disease is fairly available all over Thailand and detection of this disease is a major issue. Many recent observations identified that female are failing to admit the signs and presence of this infection and most are denying. This is resulting into refusal against the required treatment too. In fact, failing to offer needed treatment for this disease can result into major health issues down the line.

This disease can attack all age groups male and female. This disease will result into affected urethra for male to make urination difficult and paining practice. This disease will affect urethra or cervix in female and some cases experienced severe damage for both too.

This disease generally transmitted through sex, regular sex, oral sex, anal sex and through intimate contact with an individual that is already infected. There is a chance to transmit this disease to the newborns through their infected mothers too. This will result into severe eye infection or pneumonia.

Signs and Symptoms

Detecting chlamydia in the early stages is a highly impossible as symptoms will be seen absent in more than 75% cases. The symptoms will appear only after 1 to 3 weeks period after infection. Here, symptoms will be very often temporary or mild to result into missing or overlook. It is suggested consulting doctor immediately after sensing any mild symptom.

The important symptoms or signs associated with this infection are painful urination, pain at lower abdomen area, discharge from vagina, pain during sex for female, discharge through penis in male and testicular pain.

Diagnosis

It is highly essential to consider similar precautions and tests for this issue like any other STD. People with multiple sex partners, people constantly practicing unprotected sex, people with other STDs, people with sex partner that is infected with STDs should consult their doctors for immediate test procedures.

This chlamydia diagnosis requires swab culture from cervix in female and from urethra in male. There is a necessity for anus swab culture for some cases too. Here, a simple urine test can detect successfully the presence of this infection for both genders.

Treatment

There are wide varieties of antibiotics available to treat well this chlamydia. The exact treatment will mainly depend over the some special factors and doctor will be the right person to decide this treatment. Identify the real importance of advice and treatment from a professional for this disease and practice the same without fail

The two recommended treatment for chlamydia is as follows:

- Azithromycin (Azith, Zithromax) 1 g orally in a single dose.
- Doxycycline (Vibramycin) 100 mg orally twice a day for 7 days.

The single dose treatment of azithromycin may be slightly more expensive but both are considered highly effective.

Alternative regimens are:

- Erythromycin base 500 mg orally four times a day for 7 days
- Erythromycin ethylsuccinate 800 mg orally four times a day for 7 days
- Ofloxacin (Tarivid, Floxin) 300 mg orally twice a day for 7 days

- Levofloxacin  (Levaquin, Cravit) 500 mg orally once daily for 7 days

Taking treatment for chlamydia is never be enough unless practicing the same for the sex partner too. It is highly essential to keep away from sex for total seven days from the beginning day of the treatment.


**Gonorrhea:**

Gonorrhea is another serious STD results through the neisseria gonorrhoeae bacterium. This bacterium will be more rampant and improves in multiple numbers at warm and moist areas such as female cervix, reproductive tract, uterus and fallopian tubes. Similarly, it will grow well in urethra of both male and female too. This disease generally present in the areas such as throat, mouth, eyes, and anus. According to global statics, this disease is every year affecting around 62 million people worldwide. In fact, most of the cases among the affected are mild and easy to cure too. This disease is quite rampant in Thailand and resulting into a major issue. Growing sex service industry is the major reason for this crisis. Most of the sex workers are considering self-medication for this purpose through some of the antibiotics and this is making the trouble further stronger to make it hard to control.

Signs and symptoms

There is a chance for few people to witness no symptoms through gonorrhea. In fact, the symptoms will start to appear only after 14 days of the infection. The first and foremost symptom associated with this disease is burning feeling while urination. Also, there is a chance to witness yellow or white discharge in male and greenish to yellow discharge in female from anus. Men generally witness swelling in testicles with pain and female will experience bleeding during periods due to this infection.

The symptoms in female due to this infection are often mild to make the situation into wrong diagnosis as bladder or urethra infection. It is quite easy and quick to identify the symptoms in male unlike in female.

Diagnosis

The test considered for the confirmation of gonorrhea requires sample from the infected portion through a cotton swab. It is a good idea to mention with the doctor about anal sex and oral sex practice, which will consider collecting samples from throat and rectum too for the confirmation. Urine sample and testing is part and parcel of this entire diagnosis process.

Treatment

Ciprofloxacin, Ofloxacin and Levofloxacin are widely used as treatment for gonorrhea. However, since gonorrhea in Thailand has developed resistance to certain antibiotics, the Center for Disease Control (CDC) has now recommended only one class of antibiotics to treat gonorrhea. Cephalosporins are now used to treat the infection.

- Ceftriaxone (Rocephin) 250 mg single dose via intramuscular injection
- Cefixime (Cefspan, Sixime) 400 mg single dose orally
- Cefpodoxine 200 mg single dose orally
- Cefotixin (Cefoxin) 2 g single dose orally

Another option is Azithromycin (Azith, Zithromax) 1 g single dose orally. This can also cure chlamydia, which is often also found with gonorrheal infections.

It is highly essential to keep away from sex and alcohol during medication for the gonorrhea disease.

**HIV and AIDS:**

Most of the current famous developing countries are successful to have helpful health plans for their citizens including for sexually transmitted diseases. Thailand is doing significant extent for the past ten years in this context for reducing the STD severity and emphasized more over AIDS and HIV.

In the year 1984 Thailand witnessed the first case of AIDS. Currently, there are around 143,000 HIV infections in Thailand basing on the 10991 records. Thailand in this context initiated massive health program along with proper information system for their citizens. This campaign's main aim is to reduce STD, HIV and AIDS to a great extent. This action plan helped Thailand to reduce the infections up to 19,000 in the year 2003. Recently, government initiated a new condom program through targeting sex service workers in the country and making all arrangements for its adherence from the sex workers too.

The 2009 records are indicating 530,000 HIV victims in Thailand despite having proper action plan to control this disease. This kind of situation is resulting into serious advocacy towards controlling AIDS and HIV on a regular basis in Thailand.

Causes

The HIV or Human Immunodeficiency Virus capable enough to destroy CD4 cells within the body and this is a white blood cell that strives well for human immune system. These cells are widely popular as T Cells too. Destruction to T cells will results into reduced immune system for the human body. Here, HIV is a group of viruses widely known as retroviruses. A seasoned HIV infection will successfully transform into AIDS within two years span of time depending on few factors like environment, viral and host. It is a common mandatory procedure for HIV to transform into AIDS. HIV is considered as AIDS, when CD4 cell count falls to less than 200 cells/mm3. This kind of situation will result into multiple complications ranging from infection, neurologic symptoms, cancer and wasting syndrome.

Signs and Symptoms

The transformation of HIV into AIDS will vary drastically from one individual to other. In some cases more than 20 years will be required for this transformation too. The average progression period will be between 8 and 10 years, when there is no availability for antiretroviral therapy.

There is a chance for the infected person to experience variety of symptoms as acute infection within few weeks after infection. Very commonly these types of infections are described by the experts as influenza kind illness. It will range in general from fever, body pains, sore throat and glands swelling. The infected person will be completely symptoms free after the primary stage for a certain period. This period is quite dangerous as increased damage will start to happen over the infected individual's T cells through the virus. This will result into weak immune system and creates a chance for mild HIV symptoms such as fungal infections, diarrhea, chronic rashes, weight loss and fatigue. Down the line virus will destroy more CD4 cells in a way to turn the infected individual's body face severe complications of HIV like malignancies, infections, more weight loss and reduced mental function. Here is a chance to fight back this situation with the help of antiretroviral therapy. Very often this therapy helped many infected people restore health conditions to a good extent.

Diagnosis

A blood test is a wise choice when suspected having HIV infection. This test is very commonly known as ELISA or Enzyme Linked Immuno-Sorbent Assay test.

The ELISA test will help to find out the HIV antibodies and these results will be confirmed through conducting Western Blot test. The latest developments are now enabling finding HIV antibodies through testing saliva and this test hardly takes twenty minutes to complete and to announce results. There is a chance for the ELISA test to offer negative results for the infected person tested during window period or asymptomatic period. HIV infection test will be conducted to find out the antibodies presence and this test is widely popular as HIV RNA or p24. Most of the testing centers in Thailand are providing routine screening for people through these tests.

Treatment

There is no scaffolding evidence confirming treating AIDS and HIV through the currently available therapies. The treatment for this infection will be purely to improve immune system and to control the complications resulted through the disease. The therapy or medication should be considered from approved physician and followed properly, which can help to avoid complications to a great extent. The therapy for this infection should be considered keeping in mind all the long-term and short-term risks. Here, therapy options will be mainly dependent over the manifestation of the resulted complications.

**Alternative Treatments for STD**

Alternative treatments for STD in Thailand are used widely before the availability of costly drugs. These alternate treatment options are still favorites for many people due to the trusted tradition and their cost effective nature. Some of these alternate treatments will reduce the symptoms and helps well to clear issues for a certain period. There is a chance for the symptoms reappear again through these options. Tee tree oil is widely used by people as vaginal douche and is considered good treatment against the trichomoniasis. Similarly, a cold tea bag contains tannic acid to help well for soothing genital tissues. A mix of baking soda and cornstarch can heal the itching resulted through infection and suggested applying all over the infected portion. This application will helps well to dry sores and offers great relief from itching too. Milk is another proven treatment to obtain relief from pain and to improve healing.

www.ingramcontent.com/pod-product-compliance
Lightning Source LLC
Chambersburg PA
CBHW081444170526
45166CB00008B/2309